Understanding partial denture design

K. W. Tyson

BDS DDS FDS RCS Edin. Formerly Head of the Department of Prosthetic Dentistry and Consultant, Edinburgh Dental Hospital and School.

R. Yemm

BDS BSc PhD FDS RCS Edin. Emeritus Professor and Consultant, Dundee Dental Hospital and School.

B. J. J. Scott

BDS BSc PhD FDS RCS Edin. (Rest. Dent.) Senior Lecturer and Consultant in Restorative Dentistry, Dundee Hospital and School.

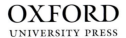

OXFORD

UNIVERSITY PRESS

OXFORD

UNIVERSITY PRESS

Great Clarendon Street, Oxford OX2 6DP

Oxford University Press is a department of the University of Oxford.
It furthers the University's objective of excellence in research, scholarship,
and education by publishing worldwide in

Oxford New York

Auckland Cape Town Dar es Salaam Hong Kong Karachi
Kuala Lumpur Madrid Melbourne Mexico City Nairobi
New Delhi Shanghai Taipei Toronto

With offices in

Argentina Austria Brazil Chile Czech Republic France Greece
Guatemala Hungary Italy Japan Poland Portugal Singapore
South Korea Switzerland Thailand Turkey Ukraine Vietnam

Oxford is a registered trade mark of Oxford University Press
in the UK and in certain other countries

Published in the United States
by Oxford University Press Inc., New York

British Library Cataloguing in Publication Data

Data available

Library of Congress Cataloging in Publication Data

Data available

Typeset by Graphicraft Limited, Hong Kong
Printed in Spain
on acid-free paper by Graficas Estella S.A.

ISBN 0-19-851092-6 (Pbk.)   978-0-19-851092-5 (Pbk.)

1 3 5 7 9 10 8 6 4 2

Foreword

In the United Kingdom, it is clear from a succession of national surveys that the oral health of the population is improving. The proportion of edentulous adults is falling significantly. There is good evidence that people are keeping their natural teeth for longer. Furthermore, with an increased life expectancy, the proportion of the population who are classified as elderly is increasing.

Although it is likely that the proportion of edentulous patients will continue to drop, this does not mean that the remainder will have intact dentitions. Loss of a few teeth may occur leaving spaces that may or may not need restoring. Some of these patients will wish to explore fixed restorations (bridges supported on the natural teeth or implants) as a means to replace teeth that have been lost. However this will not be feasible for a significant proportion of patients, particularly as they lose more teeth. For these reasons it would seem likely that the need for partial dentures is not diminishing and may even increase in the future. Alongside the retention of teeth over a much longer period other challenges may be evident. Medical conditions may affect the oral tissues. Many forms of medication may result in a reduced salivary flow which renders the teeth susceptible to further disease. The remaining teeth may be affected by toothwear or they may be in positions which are not acceptable for partial dentures. These situations will mean that great care will have to be exercised in the design of partial dentures.

The main purpose of this book is to give an understanding of the essential principles used to design partial dentures such that they will be stable in function and will not result in damage to the tissues. We have explored an approach based on an understanding of mechanical principles to introduce key concepts that should help the reader understand how to formulate suitable denture designs. We have also highlighted the important principles of designing dentures so that they are biologically favourable. An understanding of how dental plaque causes destruction of the mineralized tissues of the teeth and supporting tissues of the periodontium is outside the remit of this text. However it is critical that anyone involved in partial denture design has a sound knowledge of these disease processes. This is necessary so that the dentist can communicate in such a way so as to ensure that the patient has an insight into their susceptibility to plaque-related diseases. The patient and dentist together can institute oral hygiene regimes and maintenance to prevent further disease initiation or progression. This is especially important as even well-designed partial dentures can result in a greater susceptibility for plaque accumulation around the natural teeth. The final factor involved in good partial denture design is an understanding of the limitations of the materials themselves. This may range from using the most appropriate material for the denture base to making decisions about clasp design.

The most appropriate design of partial dentures is dependent on having good information. For this reason the dentist should be prepared to spend the time required to record a full dental, denture and medical history from the patient. It is critical that all oral tissues are examined thoroughly, both clinically and radiographically, where required. Surveyed and articulated study casts will allow the three-dimensional relationships of the maxillary and mandibular teeth to be assessed. Finally, integrated treatment plans need to be formulated to eliminate disease as well as addressing the needs of the patient by the replacement of missing teeth. Continuing advice on oral hygiene after the prostheses have been constructed should alert the patient to the potential for further disease.

The design of partial dentures should ideally be based on a team approach. It is not an activity that should be delegated to a technician nor is it one that should be in the exclusive domain of the dentist. Although the dentist has the ultimate responsibility for the patient and will therefore have the lead role, there is much to be gained by involving the technician in decisions about design at an early stage. Apart from the practical skills to fabricate the appliances, the dental technician will often have particular expertise in the limitations of the materials under certain conditions. There is therefore much to be gained from involving the dental technician, not least in that it may give an alternative design viewpoint which can be explored.

The need for well-designed partial dentures is as critical today as it has ever been. It is our hope that this book will give the reader a sound foundation, from which the principles can be applied to the wide range of clinical presentations in patients requiring partial dentures.

Contents

How to use this book

The content is divided into three distinct sections: Section 1 covers the component parts of partial dentures and the role they play in the design of a safe, functional prosthesis. It is therefore *essential* that this section be studied with care and fully understood.

Section 2 provides a sequence, or 'route map' for the process of patient examination and the decision to provide partial denture(s). The development of an appropriate design follows, using the components and their methods of function described in Section 1. In general, this section assumes the presence of a reasonably healthy, stable residual dentition.

Section 3 introduces some of the problem areas which will be encountered, such as the unhealthy mouth and the need to include consideration of other restorative work in association with design. We also provide an initial insight into some less common methods and techniques which may assist, in carefully selected cases, with the design process.

Section 1

General principles of partial dentures and how they work

This section deals with how partial dentures *work*. It is not possible to design a well-functioning and physiologically acceptable denture without a thorough understanding of the mechanisms involved.

A partial denture is a device placed into the mouth to replace lost teeth and the accompanying alveolar process. It is therefore a substitute for part of the masticatory mechanism and, as such, should become a part of that system. If the denture is not properly designed, it cannot fulfil that function.

Section 1 examines the way in which partial dentures and their components function, and provides a basis for the understanding of the requirements of the design process.

Without this understanding you cannot design a denture to work successfully within the physiological framework as a part of the masticatory mechanism.

Why should partial dentures be provided?

Are partial dentures needed to compensate for changes due to tooth loss? The case for and against partial dentures is presented together with frequently used terminology.

Why partial dentures?

Partial dentures are provided to restore facial form and masticatory function after tooth loss.

Their bio-compatibility depends on the acceptance by the body of the materials from which the dentures are constructed, the tolerance of the tissues to the denture in function and the ability of the patient to manipulate the appliances in comfort and control plaque.

The dentures should be made of materials which are inert as far as the body is concerned and the design should be such that the denture can reproduce the functions of the missing teeth. Depending on the design, dentures can be beneficial or detrimental to oral well-being.

The dentures, as mechanisms, should be constructed to fit the mouth comfortably yet carry out the functions of the missing tissues efficiently and without detriment to the remaining hard or soft tissues. They need to:

- restore form (aesthetics) and function
- restore speech and mastication
- be tissue compatible
- comfortable and well tolerated
- avoid compromising oral hygiene

Considering these points, take an overall look at the question of the provision of partial dentures. Some day, it may be that tooth loss will become such a rare occurrence that the question of replacement will no longer be an important part of general dentistry. Defeat of the most common causes of tooth loss, caries, and periodontal disease, needs not only a successful dental profession but also fundamental behavioural changes on the part of the population.

Teeth are lost—so what?

For the patient the teeth serve three main purposes, those of facial appearance, speaking, and mastication. Therefore tooth loss would result in:

- loss of appearance
- loss of clear speech
- loss of masticatory function

The presence of a natural dentition, in good order, is a socially acceptable state. Facial expression ('smile, please' for a photograph), successful and comfortable chewing in company, freedom of dietary selection, enjoyment of eating, and clear speaking are all factors which are taken for granted by an ordinary person. Tooth loss can affect one or more of these factors.

There are other consequences of tooth loss which are of less immediate impact.

The dentition functions as a whole, and if sections are destroyed the equilibrium is disturbed. The degree of disturbance is dependent on the number and position of the missing teeth. For instance there may be loss of masticatory efficiency leading to poor comminution of the food bolus and its mixing with saliva at the start of the digestive process.

Drift and overeruption

Teeth, even in adulthood, retain the ability to move within the alveolar bone. Therefore, space made by tooth extraction can allow drift and tilting of teeth mesial and distal to the space. Loss of opposing occlusion can permit overeruption. These tooth movements are slow, difficult to correct, or in most cases of overeruption, irreversible, further detracting from the integrity of the dentition and the scope for maintenance.

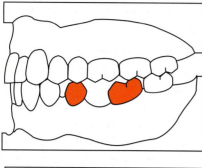

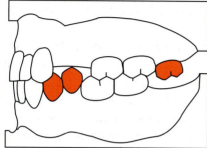

Changes in muscle and joint function

Chewing, in particular, involves complex muscle and joint movements within the head and neck. These subconscious activities can be altered by tooth loss. Adaptation is required, and may not be achieved easily, especially in older people. For instance, most people have a 'preferred' chewing side, which can be upset by tooth loss on that side.

Tooth wear

Normal function, even with modern diets, can result in gradual tooth wear. When spread over an intact dentition, this is generally so slow as to be of only academic significance. However, tooth loss concentrates this wear on the remaining surfaces and may become significantly destructive over a period. Parafunction can lead to excessive wear. Furthermore, particular dietary habits, such as the excessive intake of carbonated or some fruit beverages, may be associated with dental erosion.

The consequences of tooth loss may be:

- loss of tooth morphology
- loss of face height due to tooth wear (although this may often be compensated by overeruption, or compensatory alveolar growth, as long as there are opposing teeth)
- forward positioning of the mandible
- locking of the dentition due to opposing tooth loss or loss of vertical height
- possibility of temporomandibular joint dysfunction

Loss of occlusion

With loss of many teeth the normal relationship between maxilla and mandible, determined by the intercuspal position, can become less distinct and eventually lost. This often happens when molar and premolar teeth are lost, leaving only incisor and canine contacts. In these cases other, less precise guides to a biologically appropriate jaw relationship must be used.

The case for replacement

The patient's view:

- aesthetics
- speech
- satisfactory mastication
- should be unaware of the denture

From the patient's point of view, the replacement of lost anterior teeth is normally an essential and immediate social necessity. On the other hand from the masticatory point of view, it is remarkable how many patients claim to eat perfectly adequately yet have no posterior teeth at all.

Advantages of removable prostheses

- More teeth can be replaced
- Less interference with the remaining teeth
- Removable for cleaning
- Relatively easily repaired/replaced if there is deterioration of the teeth or dentures
- Further tooth loss is more easily managed (additions)

Disadvantages of removable prostheses

- Reduced security during function
- Must be relatively large even when replacing relatively few teeth
- The components are potentially visible (speech/smiling)
- Possibility of putting other teeth at risk (plaque/trauma)

There are clearly advantages to be gained from the replacement of lost natural teeth, provided that the process of replacement is helpful and not detrimental to the patient and also provided that function of the replacement does in fact achieve the these advantages. This text focuses on the understanding of how to design partial dentures that will be an adjunct to the patient and not to provide an appliance which will oversee the gradual destruction of what remains of the natural dentition.

Therefore only brief reference is made to fixed prosthodontics, such as bridges and implant-borne crowns. In general the latter procedures are more often restricted to patients who have lost one or a few teeth, and in whom the remaining teeth and supporting structures are sound and healthy, with good prospects for continuing self care, including avoidance of contact sports.

Replacement by a partial denture

When circumstances contraindicate a fixed replacement of missing teeth, the potential value of a removable prosthesis should be assessed. Reference to the general advantages and disadvantages, *as they relate to the individual patient*, will help to develop an appropriate strategy. In this process it may be decided that:

- all the missing teeth should be replaced
- there may be merit in replacement of some, but not all, of the lost teeth
- any replacement could do more harm than good

The benefits of partial dentures

Facial form

Loss of anterior teeth allows the lips to fall back and detract from the appearance of the patient and, if the lips are parted, there is a socially unacceptable gap on view. For the majority of patients this is intolerable. Loss of posterior teeth can, in some cases, lead to a sunken appearance of the cheeks but is not often a cause for complaint.

Function

Partial dentures should restore correct enunciation and proper function of the chewing mechanism in addition to providing improvement in food comminution, resolution of some temporomandibular joint dysfunction symptoms and prevention of glossal hypertrophy (due to the tongue taking on some masticatory function).

How can partial dentures be harmful?

- Oral hygiene
- Plaque accumulation
- Mechanical damage
- Torquing forces
- Overload

- Gingival and periodontal damage through 'gum stripping'

The principal cause for concern is that of oral hygiene. The presence of a denture in the mouth increases the risk of plaque accumulation, both on the denture itself and on adjacent natural teeth, especially if there is interference with the normal self-cleansing actions of function and saliva flow. Although it has been shown that, with meticulous oral and denture hygiene, this risk can be effectively eliminated, not all patients can be relied upon to achieve the necessary standards.

It is therefore essential to consider the oral hygiene implications of a partial denture, and to develop a design to minimize the risk of plaque accumulation and its consequences. The particular areas at risk are the gingival tissues surrounding each tooth, the interdental regions between remaining teeth, and the contact between natural teeth and denture. Tooth structure is especially vulnerable to caries when there is exposed cementum or a denture edge that lies near or over an area of gingival recession, a common feature in the older patient.

Mechanical damage can be caused to the teeth, such as through torquing forces being applied by the denture in function, abrasion of enamel or cementum by ill-fitting clasps or denture base, and by overloading teeth through the injudicious placing of occlusal rests. Soft tissue damage can be caused by, amongst other things, 'gum stripping' denture bases, poorly designed clasps and connectors applying lateral stresses to the teeth and overloading areas of mucosa used for support.

It will help therefore, if there are general guidelines, to be followed as far as possible, when designing a partial denture:

- keep the denture simple, avoiding the creation of hard-to-clean angles and crevices
- keep clear of gingival margins unless essential—leave a space of at least 3 mm between denture and gingivae wherever possible
- do not extend the denture beyond functionally justified areas

The badly damaged dentition

It is unfortunate, but true, that patients for reasons of past neglect have heavily damaged residual dentitions. The long-term prognosis for the remaining teeth may be judged to be poor, even with extreme professional and self care (and the latter often cannot be expected).

In the past, a common solution to this state of affairs was to extract the remaining teeth and provide complete dentures. A less drastic strategy, applicable to many such patients, is to provide relatively simple (and sometimes quite extensive) partial dentures as a transitional measure. Then, if and when further extractions are unavoidable, additions can be made to the dentures, which, little by little, can introduce the patient towards the manipulation of complete dentures. We will describe this option more fully in a later chapter.

DESIGN SEQUENCE

teeth to replace
support
connectors
retention
refine

We will follow these steps as we consider the design of partial dentures. We have already looked at the first point. The remainder will be examined in the sequence noted as they arise. The sequence is logical and one step leads to the next.

Conclusions

Properly designed partial dentures are an adjunct to the maintenance of oral form and function where circumstances contraindicate replacement by fixed structures. The design of any denture must be specifically tailored to the needs of that individual. **Never forget** that partial dentures should not be considered in isolation. When making a decision on whether to provide a partial denture, it is essential to have a full understanding of the patient's needs. To do this there must be a clear history of their previous denture-wearing history (if any) as well as past dental treatment. Some medical conditions make it difficult to provide dentures or make the outcome unpredictable. The condition of the remaining teeth and supporting structures of the mouth may influence how the dentures should be planned and designed. Finally the dentist needs to be reassured that the patient can reach and maintain good oral and denture hygiene.

Some points to remember

- To justify the provision of partial dentures, it must be possible to foresee continuing advantages over disadvantages
- Only replace those teeth whose loss is clearly disadvantageous

---

Note: **Principal components of partial denture**

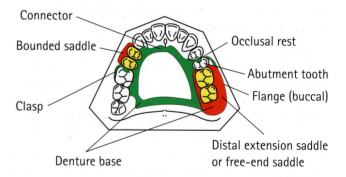

Connector
Bounded saddle
Clasp
Denture base
Occlusal rest
Abutment tooth
Flange (buccal)
Distal extension saddle or free-end saddle

Loads and levers

You cannot even begin to design a satisfactory partial denture unless you understand the essential physics involved in the workings of the appliance. Revision of these properties is therefore essential. Once understood, the development of a good design is greatly simplified.

Partial dentures are subject to many forces, such as chewing (vertical and lateral), lifting (sticky foods), and actions of the tongue, lips and cheeks. We must employ the understanding of loads and levers during the development of good design.

It could be argued that this short chapter contains the information about which the major part of this book hinges. It is purely a revision of some elementary school physics which you use daily without thinking.

Fundamental to understanding partial denture design is a solid grasp of simple mechanical principles. Without these you might as well leave the design to your laboratory or copy a design that happens to take your fancy, neither of which takes into consideration the physiological needs of the patient. The result is, rather than providing an appliance which compliments the oral tissues and masticatory mechanism, the patient is given a prosthesis which accelerates the degradation and destruction of the oral tissues. If you have taken note of the diagram with nomenclature at the end of the last chapter, you should not suddenly hit a term with which you are unfamiliar.

> If you understand how a machine works then you know **how** to use it. Similarly if you understand how a partial denture works, you will know how to approach each design problem.
>
> It so happens that the theory underlying partial denture design is **simple** if you spend a little time revising some elementary physics.

We are going to look at two essential mechanical areas, load distribution and levers.

Load distribution

Tooth support

Any load applied to a beam will be passed to the supports upon which the beam rests.

It is self-evident if the load is applied to a single support, then the full load is passed directly to that support.

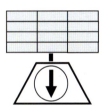

On the other hand if a load is placed centrally between two supports, the load will be divided equally between the supports. If this was applied to the saddle of a denture then the premolar would carry an equal load to the molar.

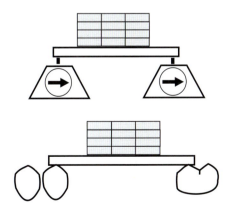

Should one support be moved further away from the load then the weight distribution would be unequal, the support nearer the load bearing more weight than the more distant support. This would be useful as a premolar, with its smaller root area, can carry less extra loading than a molar.

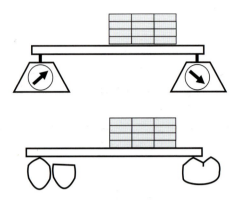

By incorporating this principle into partial denture design it is possible to see that the occlusal load on a tooth-borne saddle can be distributed to the standing teeth in proportion to their ability to withstand the extra loading.

There is however a slight complication to these simple analogies, and that is **how** the load is applied to the supports. The next diagrams show two extremes, a removable saddle with small occlusal rests on the abutment teeth and a fixed bridge. The short occlusal rests are on the edge of tapering supports and so the force is not applied to the long axes of the abutments, instead a torque is applied to these teeth.

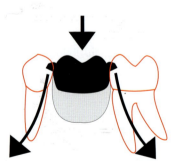

On the other hand, a bridge being like a long solid beam will apply the load vertically. You will realize that any form of occlusal rest should aim to apply the load down the long axes of the teeth to avoid damage to the periodontal ligament.

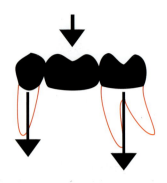

Tissue support

Loading of the soft tissues, mucoperiosteum, and mucus membrane is achieved in a different way. These tissues are not hard like the teeth so the loads are applied over as large an area as possible so that the load per unit area is reduced to a minimum.

To be functional a denture must act for the natural teeth. Occlusal and any other loading during mastication must therefore be transmitted from the denture to the foundation upon which it rests. As we know this foundation, consisting of the teeth and the mucosa, provides support for the denture.

A denture must be designed so that the supporting tissues are able to withstand the loads the denture applies to them without suffering any damage through overload or torsional stresses. In the edentulous case, where no other method of support (such as implants) is provided, we are dependent on tissue support alone.

In many large partial dentures it becomes necessary to derive support from both the teeth and the tissues to avoid overload. For example an unbounded posterior saddle will rely on tissue support as well as, anteriorly, support from the remaining teeth.

Tooth and tissue support

The difficulties, which arise when it is necessary to derive support from both the teeth and the tissues, are caused by the fact that the tissues are compressible whilst the teeth are not. This upsets the principles so far advanced as the denture would tilt, rather like the leaning tower of Pisa where one side of the foundation is softer than the other.

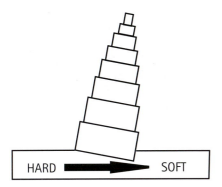

HARD → SOFT

We must also address the situation that commonly arises when a load is placed outside the supports. If you think for a moment of a free-end saddle, this only has an abutment tooth at one end, which means that only one end of the saddle can be tooth supported. If we are going to avoid introducing torsional stresses into a denture design the leverages involved must be taken into account. These stresses occur not only during occlusal loading but also in the methods by which a partial denture is retained in the mouth.

To be able to understand and overcome these difficulties, you must fully understand lever systems—something you use every day but never really think about because of common usage—the theory is simple, if understood, as is the application.

Lever systems

> 1
> The **load** is the weight or force to be acted upon.
> The **effort** is the weight or force required to cause the action.
> The **fulcrum** is the pivot about which these forces act.
>
> 2
> In a perfect system which is static:
> The effort × the distance from the fulcrum
> is equal to the load × the distance from the fulcrum.

You will remember that there are three types of lever and *around these the whole of partial denture design revolves*.

But first, three fundamental facts:

(1) A lever system works at a **mechanical advantage** when the **effort** is less than the **load**.

(2) A lever system works at a **mechanical disadvantage** when the **effort** is greater than the **load**.

(3) To be in balance (equilibrium) the forces on either side of the **fulcrum** must be equal.

That is, the effort multiplied by its distance from the fulcrum is equal to the load multiplied by its distance from the fulcrum.

> **To suit our way of thinking**
>
> The further the effort from the fulcrum the less effort needed, and equally, the nearer the load to the fulcrum the less effort needed.
>
> As in both these cases the arm of the effort lever becomes longer and the arm of the load shorter.

There are three classes of lever

Class I

The **fulcrum** lies between the **load** and the **effort**.

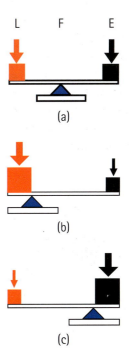

(a) Works when the load and effort are equidistant from the fulcrum. There is no mechanical advantage; the load and effort are equal.

(b) Works at a mechanical **advantage** when the load is nearer the fulcrum than the effort. The load is greater than the effort.

(c) Works at a mechanical **disadvantage** when the load is further from the fulcrum than the effort. The effort is greater than the load.

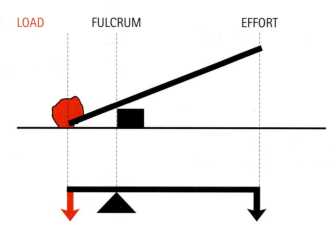

The example taken here is that of a crowbar levering a heavy rock. The greater distance of the effort from the fulcrum gives a bigger mechanical advantage.

Class II

The **load** lies between the **fulcrum** and the **effort**.

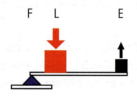

Works at a mechanical advantage. Cannot work at a mechanical disadvantage as the load is always nearer to the fulcrum.

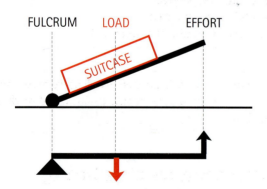

The example is a suitcase trolley where the extended handle reduces the effort by the user.

Class III

The **effort** lies between the **fulcrum** and the **load**.

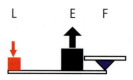

Works at a mechanical disadvantage. Cannot work at a mechanical advantage as the effort is always nearer to the fulcrum.

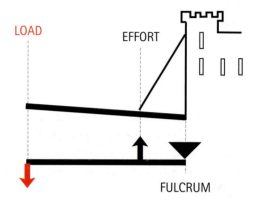

This example is a drawbridge where the effort is close to the fulcrum. This type of lever is often convenient. For example, think of the biceps muscle which has to produce about ten times the force to bend the arm when a weight is held in the hand (with the forearm horizontal). It would be more efficient but far less convenient if the lower attachment of the biceps were to be on to the wrist.

Note: **In the following chapters we will be constantly referring to these simple lever systems.**

Conclusions

You should review load distribution and how it is shared by the supports and revise the three classes of levers which are fundamental to the understanding and subsequent success of a partial denture.

Some points to remember

It is vital to grasp the theory of levers:

- the applied **load** is the biting force on the denture teeth in the case of support, or the displacing force on the denture teeth on opening when chewing sticky food
- the **fulcrum** is the point about which the denture tries to rotate
- the **effort** is the restraining component usually a clasp(s)

Classification of partial dentures

For convenience in the discussion and description of partial dentures some form of classification is useful. One which is almost universally understood is that described by Kennedy.

It is helpful to have a method of describing the type of denture required. The form and shape of partial dentures are virtually numberless, so a classification is needed to divide them into manageable groups when they are to be described or discussed.

There are two common ways of classifying partial dentures; one is based on the distribution of missing teeth saddles, the other on how the denture is to be supported. Both have merits and drawbacks. Classification by missing teeth gives an immediate mental picture of what a denture might look like but gives no indication of how the masticatory load is to be applied to the tissues. The converse applies to the classification indicating the support available. Really the two compliment each other.

The classification which is generally used is that described by Kennedy. Based on the pattern of missing teeth, it is universally understood, but gives no indication of the condition of the teeth, the supporting structures, or how the masticatory load be applied.

Note: A *bounded saddle* is an area where a tooth or teeth are missing but there is an abutment tooth at each end.

A *free-end saddle or distal extension saddle* is one where there is an abutment tooth at the anterior end only.

Third molars are frequently ignored in design discussion (being so variable) unless they have a direct use or bearing on the design under consideration.

Kennedy Classification

Class I Bilateral free-end
Class II Unilateral free-end
Class III Unilateral bounded
Class IV Anterior (*crossing the mid-line*)

The other classification is based on the way the partial denture is supported (Beckett). Here you are only given the type of support employed, not the number, distribution or condition of the missing teeth.

Classification by support

Class I Tooth supported
Class II Tissue supported
Class III Tooth and tissue supported

Reminder. A **saddle** is an area of a denture base, covering the oral mucosa, to which the artificial teeth are attached

---

Partial dentures classified by missing teeth—Kennedy

Kennedy class I

Bilateral free-end saddles

There are no teeth standing distal to the abutment teeth. Therefore the free-end or distal extension saddles can only derive tooth support at one end.

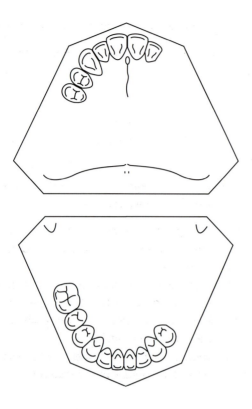

Kennedy class III

Unilateral bounded saddle

The saddle has an abutment tooth at each end; therefore the saddle could, if required, derive tooth support for the whole saddle.

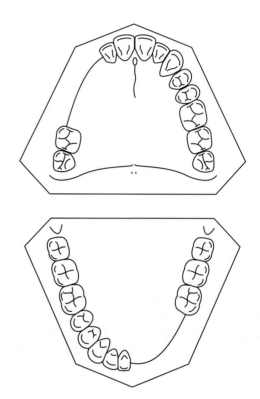

Kennedy class II

Unilateral free-end saddle

There are no teeth standing distal to the abutment tooth, therefore the saddle can only derive tooth support at one end.

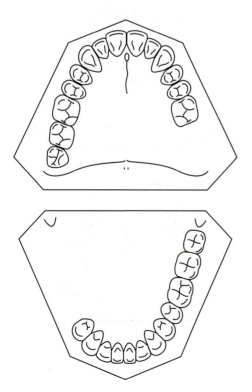

Kennedy class IV

Anterior bounded saddle (crossing the mid-line)

The anterior saddle has an abutment tooth at each end, and by definition crosses the mid-line (if it did not cross the mid-line, then it would be a unilateral bounded saddle).

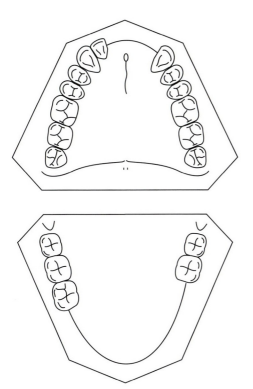

But . . . *what if there is more than one gap in an arch?*

This is taken into account by the use of **modifications to the basic classes**.

Modifications

However, matters become more complicated if there is space for more than one edentulous saddle present in an arch.

The most posterior saddle present defines the basic classification of the arch. Do **not** forget this.

Any extra saddles form *modifications* of that basic classification. The **modifications** are **numbered** according to the number of extra saddles.

For example, **three** gaps in an arch, one of which is a free-end saddle, would be a **Class II** because the most posterior saddle is a single free-end with **modification 2** because there are two other saddles.

So far so good, but there is one exception to this rule—the **Class IV** (we will deal with that separately).

This is the basis of the system which depends not on the *number* of missing teeth but from *where* they are missing.

The illustrations below show all four classes, the size of each saddle is, as we have already noted, of no consequence.

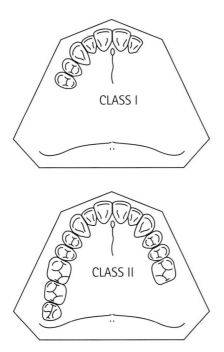

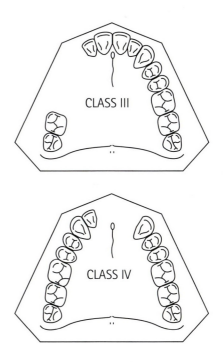

Firstly, how about trying a few examples?

What classification do you think these diagrams show?

(First decide the **classification**, then add the **modifications** if necessary.)

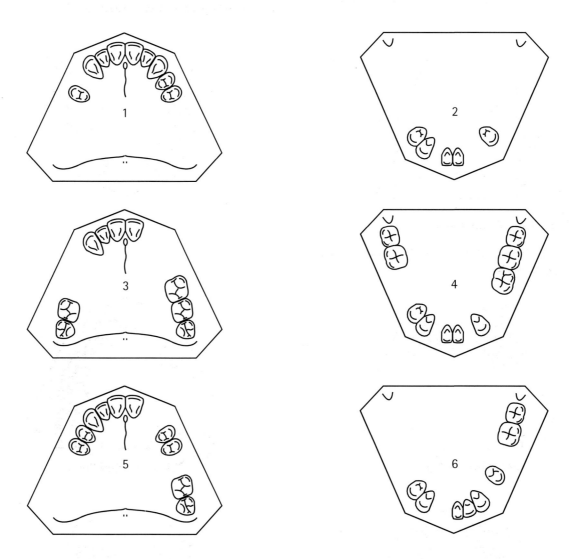

1. Class I modification 1
2. Class I modification 2
3. Class III modification 1
4. Class III modification 3
5. Class II modification 2
6. Class II modification 3

Kennedy class IV saddle

The anterior bounded saddle (crossing the mid-line) cannot have any modifications. If another saddle were present it would have to be in a more posterior position, so the **classification** would change to a I, II, or III as the most posterior saddle, by definition, decides the class.

In other words, the only time a **Class IV** classification can be used is when there is no other saddle present and it is *an anterior saddle that crosses the mid-line*.

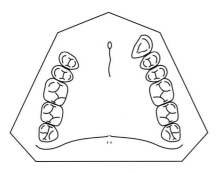

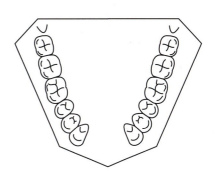

None of the next four illustrations is Class IV.

Not one of these illustrations has *only* an anterior saddle that crosses the mid-line.

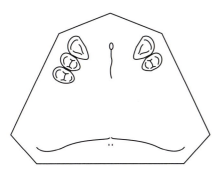

CLASS I modification 1

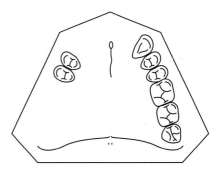

CLASS II modification 1

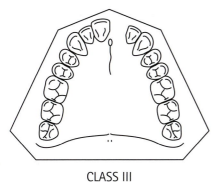

CLASS III

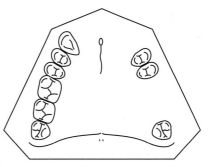

CLASS III modification 1

Try these last examples:

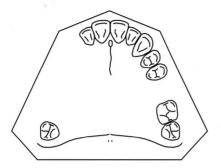

CLASS III modification 1

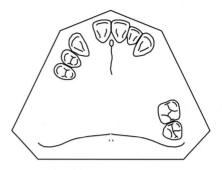

CLASS II modification 2

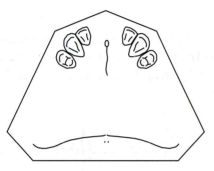

CLASS I modification 1

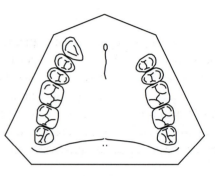

CLASS IV

That is all there is to it—a simple classification that is understood everywhere. Remember though, that no indication is given of the state of the teeth, their supporting structures or the condition of the soft tissues.

Partial dentures classified by support

This classification is very simple. It gives no indication of the number of saddles, their size or distribution, the state of the teeth and their supporting structures, and only indicates how the saddles will need to be supported.

Adding this classification to that of Kennedy gives a better idea of the partial denture under consideration.

Class I   Tooth supported
Class II   Tissue supported
Class III   Tooth and tissue supported

Therefore a Kennedy class 1, tooth and tissue supported denture tells you that the denture will have bilateral free-end saddles and will have some tooth support.

Conclusions

The most commonly used classification (Kennedy) is a means of focusing upon the general type of denture which a patient might require and is based on the missing teeth. Because of this, we will consider the types separately in the chapters of Section 2. Classification based on support is not universally used.

Some points to remember

Be sure that you have grasped:

- Kennedy class I: two free-end saddles
- Kennedy class II: one free-end saddle
- Kennedy class III: a bounded saddle
- Kennedy class IV: one anterior saddle, crossing the mid-line

Classes I, II and III can have additional bounded saddles (modifications) whereas Kennedy class IV cannot for it will become a class I, II or III.

Cast surveying

You cannot begin to design a partial denture without first surveying the casts to demonstrate undercut areas. Such areas need to be eliminated to insert/remove the denture or used to aid retention.

Surveying is an essential step in the design and construction of partial dentures. The surveying instrument draws lines on a cast so that the dentist can be sure that no rigid part of a partial denture lies in an undercut in relation to the path of insertion and removal of the appliance. An undercut is the area below the greatest diameter of a tooth, similar to the area below an overhanging cliff edge (arrowed).

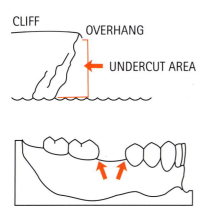

If there were undercuts present and the denture constructed to fit them, then the denture could not be fitted, or if it were forced into position, it would snap into place and be very difficult, painful or even impossible to remove (sometimes referred to as an 'insertional interference').

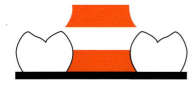

We must also find where to put clasps to hold the denture in place and how to make the prosthesis blend naturally with the tissues by avoiding unsightly gaps where the denture and tissues meet.

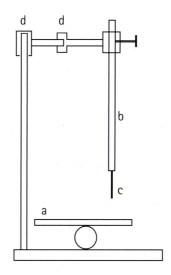

The diagram above shows the construction of a cast surveyor.

It has:

- a table (a), the angle of which can be adjusted
- a movable arm (b) carrying
- a marker lead (c) which is always held vertical by
- special joints (d)

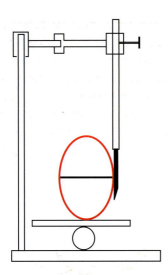

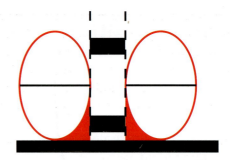

These three drawings show how this applies to a denture base:

If an object, e.g. an egg, is placed on the table and the vertical marker lead drawn around its edge, the widest part in the horizontal plane will be marked. Anything below this line is in an undercut area,

The drawn line is called the **survey line** and the area below this line is the **undercut area**, while the area above is called the **non-undercut area**.

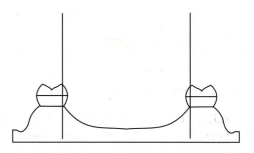

The vertical lines show the width between the necks of the teeth, and the survey lines show the level of the minimum distance available between the teeth.

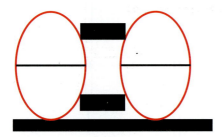

From this diagram, it is quite obvious that the upper block cannot move downward or the lower block upward.

Only something with the same width (or less) as the narrowest part between the eggs (indicated by the survey lines) could move into the undercut area from above or vice versa.

A denture base has to be inserted and removed. This is accomplished by making the base so that it cannot extend into an undercut area. If the undercut areas are removed by adding plaster of paris (shown in **red**), and a block is made to this width, it would pass upward and downward between the eggs without difficulty.

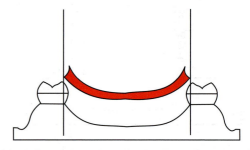

A denture base made to the width between the gingival margins (necks of the teeth) would not go into place.

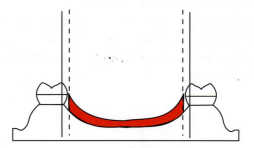

However, where the base is made only as wide as the minimum distance between the teeth, the base can be inserted and removed. So, any undercuts must be eliminated if a base is to be inserted or removed properly.

Let us have a closer look at the elimination of undercuts. The lead on the surveyor is usually sharpened to a chisel point, so that a second line appears on the cast vertically below the one on the tooth. The marker and scribed lines are shown in red for clarity.

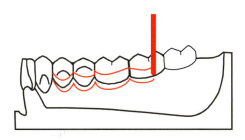

The result is that the complete undercut area is outlined. Such areas can be filled with plaster which is trimmed with a knife attached to the surveyor arm (see the next diagram) so eliminating the undercut areas in the vertical plane, *on the cast*.

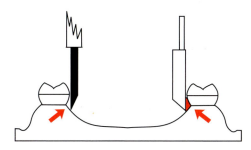

This coronal view shows the marking lead (left) and the plaster trimmer (right) indicating the undercut areas displayed and blocked out (arrowed). The knife on the right has correctly trimmed the plaster of paris.

It is essential to bring the denture base up to the survey line (below left) or there will be a space (arrowed right) *in the mouth*, resulting in a loose fitting base and a food packing area.

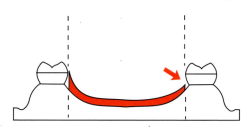

Tissue supported bases must *not* be brought above the survey line as they sink into the tissues under load. The resultant downward movement will place a lateral force on the tooth (arrowed) as the wider part moves down. (It has probably occurred to you that if the teeth withstand the lateral thrust, then the denture base must flex. This could lead to a flexural fatigue followed by fracture of the denture base.)

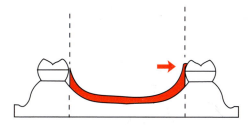

That is enough about the fit of the denture base for the moment.

We will now turn to simple retention by clasps.

Back to the eggs again. You can see that if a metal ring of smaller diameter than the egg is placed on top of the egg, it cannot pass down into the undercut area—not without a tragedy anyway.

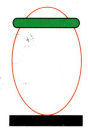

However if the ring is split, it can spring open to pass over the greatest diameter to lie passively in the undercut area. It will, of course, resist upward removal, the resistance dependent upon its springiness and the amount it has to open.

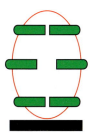

This is the principle used in making retainers or clasps which are attached to a denture base to keep it in place by engaging undercuts on the teeth.

Apply this example to partial denture retention. A typical retainer is a circumferential, occlusally approaching three-armed cast metal clasp. This translated means it goes round the tooth, goes towards the undercut from the occlusal part of the tooth, has three components, and is made of cast metal.

The three parts are the **occlusal rest** to carry the load and two tapering **arms** to retain and stabilize the denture.

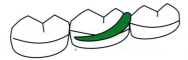

The thicker and so stiffer parts of the arms next to the rest give a bracing action against lateral thrusts.

The middle part of an active arm crosses the survey line (maximum width of the tooth) and the final third of the arm, being thinner and so springier, is the retentive part, lying passively in the undercut area where it will resist upward displacement.

So far, we have considered undercuts only in relation to the vertical plane.

We have eliminated undercuts to allow denture bases to be inserted and removed. We have talked about springing clasp arms into undercut areas to hold a denture in place.

What we have not yet considered is the fact that the teeth are not all conveniently egg shaped, that is to say, teeth vary in the curvature of their surfaces . . . so we must think about the magnitude of an undercut not only in the **vertical** plane, but also in the **horizontal** plane.

You can see the difference in shape below the survey line.

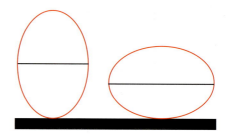

For the same depth of **vertical** undercut a clasp arm would have to be much, much springier to keep in contact with the surface on the right.

The amount of horizontal undercut that can be engaged by a clasp arm depends on the type of metal used for the clasp. For example, stainless steel wire is more able to withstand flexing than cast cobalt chromium alloy, so it can spring into (and out of) greater undercuts in the horizontal plane.

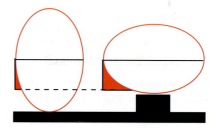

We must therefore have some way of measuring the horizontal component of an undercut, so let us consider **undercut gauges**.

We do know that the flexibility (springiness) of a wire is also dependent on its length as well as its shape and area in cross-section, but this is not at issue at the moment (see the section on clasping in Chapter 1.7).

Undercut gauges

An undercut gauge consists of a metal rod ending in a small disc. When the gauge is fitted in the chuck of a surveyor, the rod is held vertical and the disc will project sideways.

Depending on the diameter of the disc, the rod will take up different positions if both the rod and disc touch the egg at the same time. There are normally three gauges; you can see the difference in using a large and a small disc.

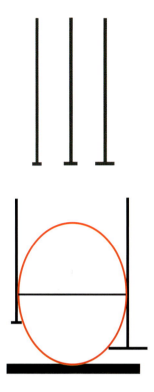

Here is the same gauge, applied to two teeth with differing buccal contours, which indicates the exact place where the horizontal undercut is correct for the flexibility of the clasp material you have chosen.

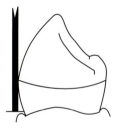

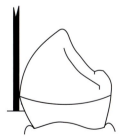

Let us look at this in greater detail.

This diagram can give you some idea of the point at which the tip of a clasp might be placed, depending on its properties.

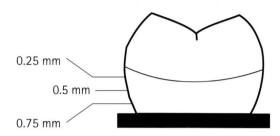

Cobalt chromium alloy is not very flexible, so a clasp tip is placed in an undercut of 0.25 mm horizontal 'depth'. Gold alloy being more flexible can employ a horizontal depth of 0.5 mm. Stainless steel wrought wire clasps, on the other hand, can happily spring in and out of undercuts of 0.75 mm depth.

As you can imagine, a cobalt chromium clasp made at 0.75 mm depth would be permanently deformed (or damage the tooth) if forced into place, whereas a stainless steel clasp at 0.25 mm would be very easily displaced and so give little in the way of retention.

All the work we have been considering so far has been with the cast lying flat, that is with the occlusal plane horizontal. This is as it should be because most of the forces tending to displace the denture are vertical—such as opening the jaws after biting into sticky foods. Unfortunately, although this is good for retention it may cause an aesthetic disaster, so we may have to insert the denture at a different angle.

Let us see why: if the cast is surveyed horizontally, you can see the undercuts on the mesial side of the canine and the anterior ridge.

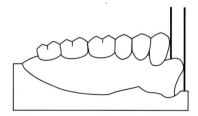

When these undercuts are blocked out so that the finished denture can be inserted and removed, there will be a space between the canine and the lateral incisor; this will look bad, and further, the flange will not fit properly against the soft tissues. This can be aesthetically, unacceptable.

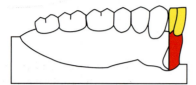

These awkward undercuts can be 'eliminated' if the table on the surveyor is tilted so that the anterior of the cast is raised. You can now see that a denture could be inserted and removed in this direction leaving no unsightly gaps.

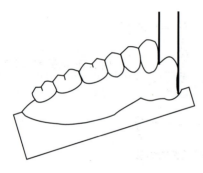

Further, the flange tucks neatly into the neck of the canine so that the lost interdental papilla and resorbed alveolus can be restored. Check this appearance with the previous diagrams.

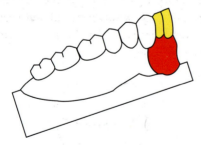

Tilting a cast can alter the apparent size of undercuts. Look at the next diagrams to see the effect of changing the angulation of the occlusal plane from the horizontal.

All the undercuts we are examining by tilting the surveyor table are related to the vertical plane.

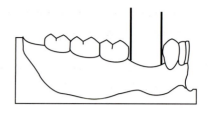

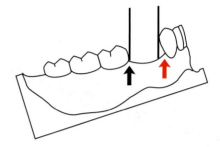

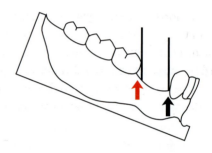

Here are three different positions of a cast. You can see that the size of the undercuts on the molar and canine can, from the vertical, be increased (**red** arrows) or reduced (**black** arrows).

Of course this also applies if a cast is tilted laterally instead of antero-posteriorly, in which case the buccal and lingual undercuts are altered.

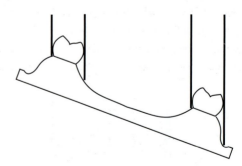

So far everything has been straightforward:

- we can use the surveyor to make sure a denture base can fit
- we can decide where to place the arms of clasps, and
- we can make a perfect blend between dentures and tissues

By now you probably expect something to upset this idyllic state, and you are not wrong.

Let us look at the situation where the sides of the abutments are at right angles to the occlusal plane.

Surveying on a tilted path gives a survey line showing undercuts.

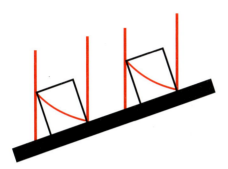

However, a horizontal survey shows that there are **no undercuts in the vertical plane** so clasps would be useless to prevent displacement of the denture in function. In other words there would be no resistance to displacement in the plane at right angles to the occlusal plane—sticky food would just lift the denture as the jaws were opened.

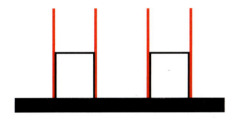

So what can we do to avoid this happening?

We must always survey a cast horizontally first, that is to find the undercuts which can be used to resist movement in the **path of displacement**. After this, if required for other reasons such as aesthetics, the cast can be tilted and surveyed again for the path of **insertion and removal**.

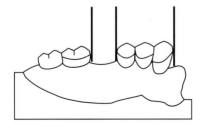

This illustration shows the markings made by a horizontal survey. The undercuts can be used for clasping to resist movement of the denture in the path of displacement.

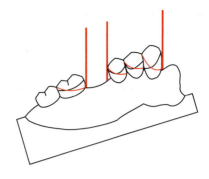

The second survey line is at a tilted path, the angle chosen here is to eliminate the undercut in the path of insertion and removal.

Does this matter?

It certainly does . . . we have now defined two areas of undercut on the teeth (which overlap). Different coloured leads are usually used to avoid confusion.

PATH OF DISPLACEMENT

PATH OF INSERTION/REMOVAL

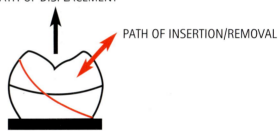

Clasp tips placed under the **black line** (horizontal survey) will resist movement at right angles to the occlusal plane and so resist displacement when the jaws open after biting into sticky food.

Clasp tips placed under the **red line** will resist movement in the line of insertion/removal and keep the denture steady in that path (usually chosen, you remember, to avoid poor aesthetics).

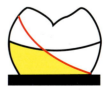

If the tip of a clasp is placed into the area where the two undercuts overlap it will resist movement in both the paths of displacement and insertion/removal.

Look at this in detail . . . the area above **both** survey lines presents no undercuts at all. The area under the **red** line (A+C) is undercut in relation to the tilted path. The area under the **black** line (B+C) is undercut in relation to the horizontal path. The undercut area common to both surveys is the **yellow** area (C).

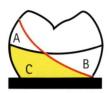

The tips of the clasps must be placed into this common undercut area to retain the denture properly.

It is only in this way that the denture will resist movement in both the path of displacement and the path of insertion/removal.

Do you understand this? If not work on it, or ask—it is absolutely vital.

We have agreed that the common undercut area is the place to put the tip of a clasp if a denture is to be retained in the paths of displacement and insertion/removal. But there is more . . .

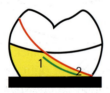

Remember that the tip of a clasp can only be placed so far into an undercut consistent with its flexibility. In this case the tip must lie somewhere on the **green** line 1–2, at the correct horizontal 'depth' below the insertion/removal survey line, so that it can flex properly as the denture is inserted and removed from the mouth. A further point to keep in mind is the length and flexibility of the arm engaging the undercut, short clasp arms can have too little flexibility.

But note this and note it well.

At position 1 resistance to vertical displacement and to insertion/removal will be about equal, but the further towards position 2 the tip is placed, the deeper it will be in relation to the horizontal undercut of the path of displacement. This is exactly what we want, as the resistance to displacement during function will be greatly increased (there is, of course, a danger of forced displacement vertically that could distort a clasp arm).

Further considerations

We have been talking a lot about clasps, but now it is time we got back to the denture base again.

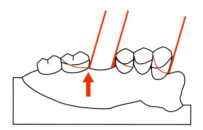

In this illustration, the cast has been surveyed to give a path of insertion along the **red** lines. The undercut on the canine has been eliminated. The **black** line on the molar shows that the denture base will be in the undercut *in the path of displacement*. What could be better? That part cannot be displaced vertically.

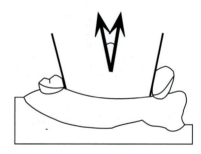

On the other hand things can become more difficult if the abutments are divergent. You can see that in the path of displacement, the base can be removed at any angle between the diverging lines. Clasping must be so arranged as to prevent such movement within this **zone of displacement**.

Zones of displacement **can be created artificially**. The next diagram shows that with minimum blocking out, there is a single path of displacement to be resisted.

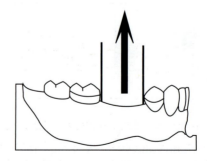

Here the cast has been surveyed again at an arbitrary angle for insertion/removal.

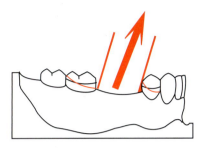

Blocking out both sets of undercuts produces a zone of displacement to be resisted. In this case, where there is no anterior saddle to create problems with aesthetics, a double survey is unnecessary. Not only unnecessary but also bad planning as the problems of retention have been increased by producing a zone of displacement.

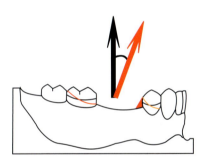

Another factor we must remember to keep in mind is that of the free-end saddle. As this type has an abutment at one end only, it is possible for the denture base to move backwards, away from that tooth (unless this is prevented by some other part of the denture base).

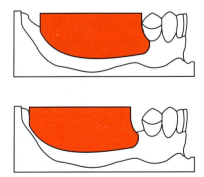

Of course this can be prevented by designing components such as a lingual plate which engages the lingual embrasures of the standing teeth or by mesial occlusal rests. Nonetheless the zones of displacement must be considered, for as we have seen, the greater the zone of displacement the more efficient must be the clasping.

Consider the following illustrations.

These diagrams illustrate the free-end saddle situation.

A vertical survey in the path of displacement makes a zone of displacement throughout a right angle.

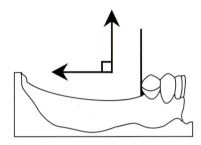

Raising the anterior of the cast to make a downward and backward path of insertion increases the zone of displacement.

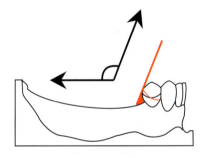

Raising the posterior of the cast gives the smallest zone, and further, allows the distal undercut on the abutment tooth to be used to resist upward displacement. This is altogether the best solution (provided there is no anterior saddle to cope with).

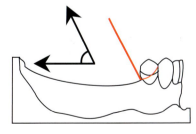

Lastly, do not be blinded by all the straight paths that appear to be shown by the surveyor. Indeed, the common surveyors can only indicate straight paths.

Certain rotational paths of displacement may develop due to the morphology of the teeth. Look at the next diagram.

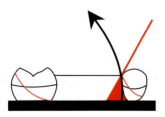

You can see that the distal undercut on the premolar has been blocked out (**red**) to allow an angled path of insertion. The mesial undercut on the molar, under the **black** line, will resist vertical displacement.

However, the curvature of the mesial surface of the molar may allow the denture base to act as a hinge, so that the anterior part of the saddle can displace upwards and backwards. The greater the tilt of the cast the greater the zone of displacement; take account of this in your clasping.

We have completed the major part of surveying.

We are now left with undercuts relating to soft tissues.

This illustration shows the soft tissue undercuts which have to be blocked out for posterior lingual flanges to insert when there are instanding molars.

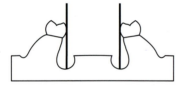

Here is the area to be blocked out if a buccal flange is not to traumatize the undercut tuberosity on insertion/removal.

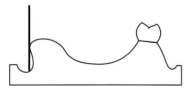

Although the resilience of the soft tissues will allow small undercuts to be engaged, larger bilateral undercuts must be eliminated.

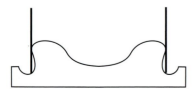

Unilateral undercuts need not always be removed as the denture can sometimes be slipped in at an angle.

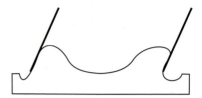

Do realize though that it is all common sense. If you are still puzzled about anything, now is the time to ask someone about it. Like so many things, once you understand something, the problems go away—or recede considerably at least.

Just a useful little tip to finish with, when you are first looking at a cast you can replace the marking lead with a metal **analysing rod**. This lets you examine the undercuts present and the various tilts you may think of selecting, without making confusing marks on the cast.

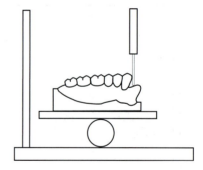

Once you are happy with your examination, carry on and mark the cast with the black and red leads.

However do not forget to draw reference lines, using the surveyor lead, on the cast to show its orientation in the surveyor in the path of insertion/removal (the path of displacement is optional as the table and cast are then horizontal). This is helpful to record the orientation of the cast in the path of insertion/removal should it have to be removed from the surveyor, to be remounted at a later time.

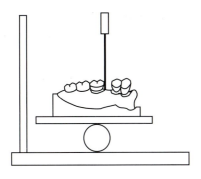

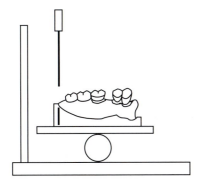

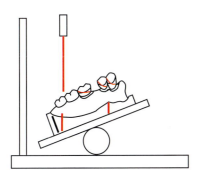

Conclusions

A cast is surveyed to show:

- undercut areas in the path of displacement of a denture
- undercut areas in the path of insertion/removal, which may or may not be the same as the path of displacement
- the best path of insertion of a denture for aesthetic and retentive purposes
- undercuts to be employed for clasps or other retentive devices
- assessment of soft tissue undercuts

Some points to remember

Surveying of accurate study casts is essential:

- for the identification of possible paths of insertion/removal and displacement of a denture
- to show where potential sources of retention are located, for clasps or by selection of a favourable path of insertion into an undercut zone

1.5 Support

Support comes from the foundation upon which a denture rests. A denture must therefore derive support from the teeth, tissues or a mixture of both. Due to the difference in compressibility of the periodontium and the mucoperiosteum under load, the tooth and tissue supported denture raises problems.

DESIGN SEQUENCE

teeth to replace
support
connectors
retention
refine

The first question we should ask is how do the teeth and mucosa support the denture, after all, the remaining teeth have only supported themselves in the past and the mucosa is not well adapted to withstand masticatory loads.

The mucosa or really the mucoperiosteum covering the residual ridges, although not accustomed to carrying occlusal loads, can withstand reasonable intermittent loading. The policy here, then, is to cover as great an area as possible with the denture base to spread the load, so reducing the load per unit area on the tissues.

> **Useful rules of thumb**
>
> A healthy tooth can withstand its own occlusal loading plus that of one and a half similar teeth.
>
> If soft tissue is to provide support then cover the greatest possible area. Reduction of the occlusal area will also reduce the load required to penetrate a bolus.

Let us look at tooth support first

It is generally accepted that each healthy standing tooth has enough spare capacity to carry not only its own loading but that of one and a half **similar** teeth. The word 'similar' is essential, you could hardly ask a lower lateral incisor to carry the load of its adjacent canine and half the first premolar—it has such a small root area that its departure would be hastened.

Occlusal rests

Occlusal rests are usually made of metal to transfer the load from a partial denture to the teeth.

Any rest placed on the occlusal surface of a tooth:

- must not cause damage to that tooth or the supporting structures
- must not interfere with the occlusion and be no less than 0.5 mm thick
- must apply the force down the long axis of the tooth with no torque

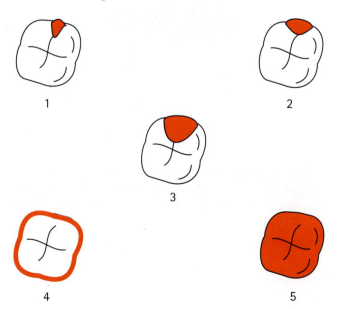

Various rests placed on the occlusal surface of a molar tooth

Small rests (1) and (2) apply large forces per unit area and may damage the enamel. Larger rests (3) cover more enamel and can direct the forces down the long axis of the tooth better.

It follows then, that a ring rest (4) is even better, and if you take this to its logical conclusion the best possible rest would be a full surface coverage (5). If a rest is to be placed on a restored tooth, care should be taken to ensure that the additional load can be withstood by the restoring material.

Small rests should be avoided as they tend to apply torsional forces to the abutment teeth. They should cover enough of the occlusal surface to direct loads axially. Of course, the best is by way of a ring rest, occlusal coverage, or a crown; this was discussed under 'loads and levers'. You will remember this illustration.

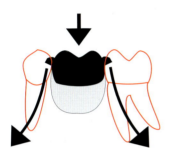

Small rests, poorly directing occlusal loading

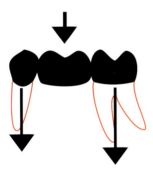

Fixed bridge directing forces down the long axes

Try to load the teeth axially, cingulum rests cut into the enamel of anterior teeth are, due to the thin enamel layer, best restricted to the canines and should be cut with the greatest care.

Rests cut into the enamel of the cingulum can direct the applied load down the long axis of the tooth

Incisal rests or embrasure hooks may be useful but can be aesthically poor, and for this reason are not often used.

Preparations for embrasure hooks or incisal rests

The masticatory pressures are intermittent, and the rest or plate prevents other lateral forces, so that the teeth are unlikely to move or otherwise come to harm unless they are very heavily loaded.

Tooth supported prostheses

We should now look at how the loads applied to the teeth by a partial denture can be distributed to the greatest advantage. Keep in mind that load distribution is a matter of simple mechanics (which sometimes might not be clinically acceptable, such as in the case of incisal rests which can be visible).

So far we have explored how the teeth can be loaded. Let us now see how the load can be distributed.

Each set of diagrams shows three representations of the same situation: a loaded beam on supports, below which is a sketch of a saddle supported by teeth and finally, at the bottom, a partial denture.

Consider these examples, **just looking at the mechanics** of load distribution.

Scenario 1

In this first case the load is distributed equally between the supports, that is to say the premolar and molar each carry half the occlusal load. This is satisfactory for a short saddle, but a longer saddle might lead to overloading of the premolar.

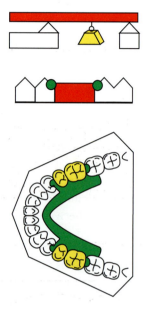

Scenario 2

By moving the anterior support further away from the load, the load on that support becomes less while increasing the load on the posterior support. Here then the premolar carries less of the load than the molar, so the length of saddle is not so critical before the premolar becomes overloaded.

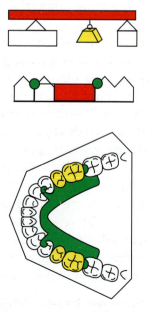

Scenario 3

If the left support is moved yet further away, the loading becomes even less on the anterior tooth (canine) but the loading on the molar is becoming rather large.

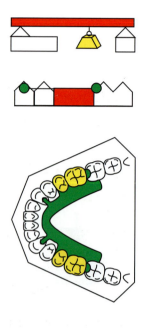

Scenario 4

Of course there is no reason why there should not be multiple supports, here both the premolar and canine share their part of the load.

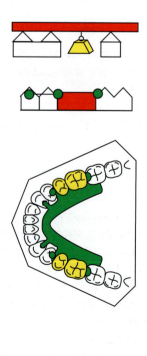

Scenario 5

In this case you are almost back to square one again. Moving the molar rest to the distal side of the tooth will result in the canine and molar sharing the load equally.

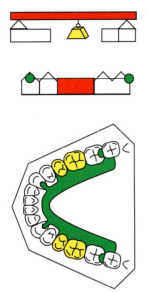

In clinical practice, it is common for scenario 1 to be used for short saddles.

By planning the distribution of the rests you can adjust the way in which the occlusal load applied to tooth supported saddles is carried by the standing teeth. Keep in mind that a healthy tooth can carry its own load plus that of one and a half **similar** teeth. The loading of tooth supported saddles is quite straightforward as you have seen. However it is a very different situation when a saddle can only be supported at one end by the teeth. Before entering into that minefield we will have a look at the possibility of partial dentures which are supported by the soft tissues only.

Tissue supported partial dentures

Total tissue support would be achieved in the absence of **any** occlusal or cingulum rests, and without **any** components contacting teeth above the survey line. In such a case, tissue loading would have to be minimized by maximum extension of the denture base to reduce the load per unit area, and also by reducing the size of the occlusal table (by using narrow buccolingual diameter teeth or by leaving off the last molars).

However, even with these precautions, there are some other problems, essentially stemming from tissue displacability (often called tissue compression).

First, every time occlusal load is applied, the denture will be driven into the tissues, and the saddles will impinge upon adjacent gingival margins, creating the classic 'gum stripper'.

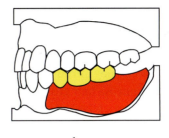

1

All teeth in occlusion no loading

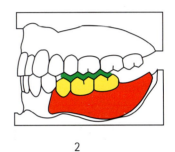

2

Tissue supported saddle loaded

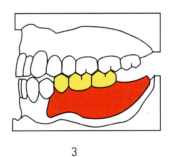

3

Artificial teeth meet first

Second, if there are natural tooth contacts, these will arrest jaw closure before tissue loading can contribute fully (1), so that the bolus is incompletely penetrated (2), unless there is premature contact with the tissue supported saddle (3). In other words, under masticatory load a tooth may be intruded into its socket by about 0.1 mm whereas the mucosa can be compressed by up to 2 mm in places. This really means that the artificial teeth should meet just before the natural teeth in the chewing areas, so that the soft tissues are well compressed before the natural teeth finally meet.

While this last is a theoretical possibility, achievable when recording jaw relationships or the impression under 'compressive' loading, in practice tissue adaptation, possibly by bone remodelling, will soon negate the attempt.

Such clinical issues can become complex and are frequently the subject of debate.

Tooth and tissue supported prostheses

We have made reference more than once to the difference in 'compressibility' of the teeth and the soft tissues under load since the teeth may intrude about 0.1 mm into their sockets and the mucosa may give way by up to 2 mm.

You have seen that it is fairly simple to deal with dentures which are supported by either the teeth or the tissues on their own.

> The foundation of a tooth and tissue supported denture is partly unyielding and partly yielding as in the Kennedy class I and II situation. Therefore the denture may tend to rock.

Mixing the two forms of support is not so easy as it appears at first sight.

If you look at a partial denture as a rigid structure with one part of it lying on the teeth and another part of it lying on the mucosa, then its foundation is partly uncompressible and partly compressible. If this denture is loaded then it will not be stable. Let us take a simple mechanical example of this situation.

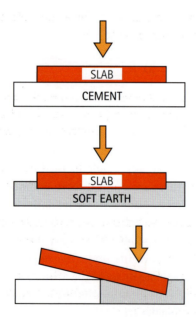

A paving slab lying on a uniform foundation will spread the applied load and remain as it is or sink a bit depending on the solidity (compressibility) of the foundation.

Clearly, as in the third diagram, where the foundation is made of dissimilar materials, the **slab will rock about the edge of the most unyielding substance**.

Note this well, as this is exactly what happens with partial dentures that have a rigid, unyielding denture base. There is more give in the soft tissues than the teeth, so when a denture is supported by both the teeth and the tissues, the denture **will rock about the occlusal rest nearest the tissue supported part of the denture when the tissue supported part is loaded**.

Apply this to a denture. A load applied to the centre of a completely tissue supported saddle will cause it to compress the tissues evenly.

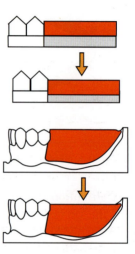

Next is a representation of a free-end saddle that has an occlusal rest at one end. You can see the result of loading. The tissue supported area sinks as the tissues compress but the distal surface of the second premolar takes a tremendous amount of weight and a distal twist.

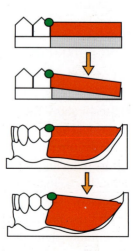

In this case we are dealing with a rest that is next to a tissue supported saddle. The situation is clinically and mechanically bad—too much load and torque on the abutment tooth.

What can be done about it? . . . Go back to simple mechanics again (you always have to).

Try moving the occlusal rest further away from the saddle.

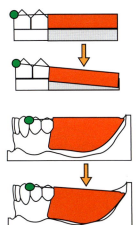

That is better, as there is not too much load applied to the first premolar and a more even compression of the tissues behind the second premolar.

You can also see that the torque is less and furthermore the rest is applied mesially to a tooth that has another one helping to stabilize it from behind; altogether much better mechanically. It is, however, common practice to place the rest on the mesial side of the premolar adjacent to the saddle.

Fine—but why not add on a few more rests to spread the load on to even more teeth? Sure, but if you look at

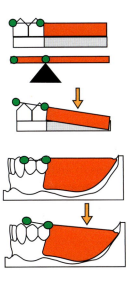

the mechanics involved, it will not help in the slightest. Think about it for a moment (for example adding a rest distally on the second premolar). If you do this, the distal rest now becomes the fulcrum.

The result is that any part of the denture base in front of that rest will lift when the saddle is loaded.

Of course this means that **any rest that is anterior to the most distal rest will be useless for support**—remember how the paving slab rocked on the edge of the concrete part of its foundation as the part over the soft earth sank?

(Do keep in mind that such extra rests might be used as indirect retainers, to be considered quite separately from support in tooth and tissue supported partial dentures.)

Conclusions

- When considering denture support, beware of causing damage to teeth or periodontal tissues by excessive loading.
- Rests must be sufficiently large but not interfere with the occlusion.
- A healthy tooth will carry its own load plus one and a half **similar** teeth.
- Occlusal forces must, as far as possible, be directed down the long axes of teeth.

Some points to remember

- Occlusal rests should be 0.5 mm minimum thickness and be sufficiently large to spread and direct the occlusal load, as far as possible, down the long axes of the teeth
- Cingulum coverage should be over at least half the tooth, and rest seats be approached with the greatest care
- Sound teeth (with sound supporting structures) can normally carry their own load plus the load of one and a half **similar** teeth
- Placement of rests requires thought as to the mechanics involved, otherwise they may not serve their expected purpose
- Tissue supported dentures must not contact teeth at any point above the survey line
- Tooth and tissue supported prostheses rest on a foundation of variable compressibility

1.6 Connectors

Connectors hold the various parts of a denture together. Major connectors join the saddles while minor connectors join smaller elements such as clasps and occlusal rests to the denture base.

Rigid connectors

Once you have decided on the teeth you are going to replace, and how the saddles are to be supported, it is time to determine how you are going to join the saddles together. In this section we are going to deal with rigid connectors which will hold the parts of the denture together without distortion.

DESIGN SEQUENCE

teeth to replace
support
connectors
retention
refine

The first paragraph is not just stating the obvious, anterior teeth certainly will be replaced but not always posteriors. For example, why replace a missing last molar that has no opponent—it will serve no purpose and may complicate the design.

On the other hand there might be a standing last molar in the upper jaw, which could over-erupt and cause problems with the occlusion unless you provide it with an opponent, so replacement is indicated.

Connectors are divided into broad categories, **major** and **minor**

Major connectors join saddles together and form the structure of the denture base.

Minor connectors are used to join smaller components, such as occlusal rests and clasps, on to the denture base.

Let us look at upper dentures first (we are only looking at the connectors).

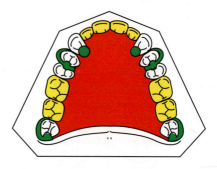

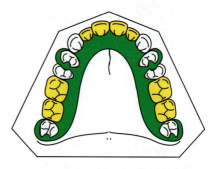

Denture bases made of plastic materials such as acrylic resin have to cover a large part of the palate to be strong enough to withstand functional stresses. Metal-based dentures though can be made as a skeleton 'base' leaving much of the palate uncovered.

See the box at the end of this chapter to compare the denture base materials.

The gingival margins should either be covered, or preferably cleared by at least 3 mm. Anything less than 3 mm can lead to food packing and stagnation (another nasty thing that can happen to small spaces is that the soft tissues can enlarge into the gap).

Palatal bars

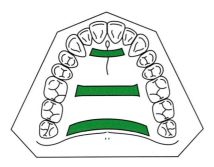

There are several ways to join the parts of an upper denture. This diagram shows (separated) **palatal bar connectors**

- **anterior palatal bar**
- **middle palatal bar**
- **posterior palatal bar**

The next diagram shows an **anterior palatal plate** (a horseshoe design).

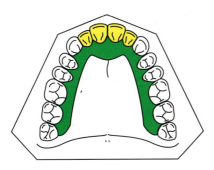

This can also be used in combination with palatal bars. Much depends on the strength required and the way the patient is able to handle (or more likely mishandle) the denture. It is always preferable to keep the incisive papilla area uncovered if possible.

There follows some major connectors joining bilateral bounded saddles (**Kennedy class III** modification 1).

The **anterior palatal bar** (a type of 'horseshoe' design), shown in the diagram, is clear of the incisive papilla. Wide, thin bars are better tolerated than narrow thick bars.

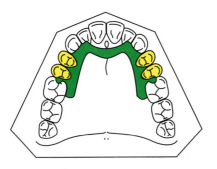

Next is a **middle palatal bar**. The advantage of this design is that a large area in the incisive papilla region is left open—this is much appreciated by many patients. The posterior part of the palate is also completely free.

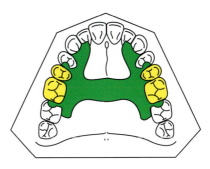

The **posterior palatal bar** is set back to the anterior border of the vibration or 'ahh' line, it is broad and thin, as are all palatal bars. The greater part of the palate is not covered and it can be well tolerated by some patients, unless the patient has an easily triggered gagging reflex.

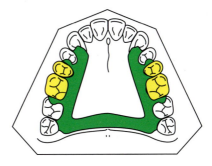

Here is an example of a **Kennedy class IV** denture.

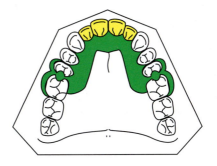

Either cover, or preferably clear, the gingival margins. The incisive papilla area in this case has to be covered, as it is the incisors which are being replaced.

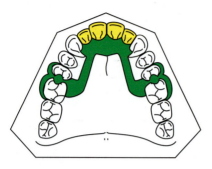

In this illustration you can see that the gingival margins have minimal coverage. The margins are cleared by at least 3 mm to avoid problems of stagnation or tissue hypertrophy. There is no loss of efficiency as far as the denture is concerned as the load is still carried by the canines, the clasping system is not compromised and the connectors are clear of the gingival margins.

Let us go back for a moment to the acrylic versus cast base question.

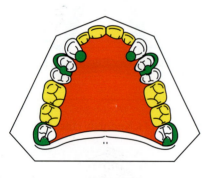

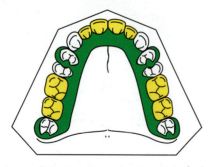

These cases are identical. It is difficult with these multiple saddles to clear the gingival margins in the canine/premolar regions, as the space left open would be too small to be effective (remember, you should always arrange the denture base to leave a tooth in a self-cleansing area, never in an interdental embrasure where stagnation will occur).

The greater strength of the metal base lets you expose the palate. If the base is not strong enough and the patient is heavy handed, then a posterior palatal bar would have to be added (sometimes called a 'ring connector').

Lower connectors

So much for the upper, for the moment, however the same principles apply to lower dentures:

- strength
- avoid gingival trauma
- keep tissue coverage to a minimum
- avoid areas allowing food packing or tissue hypertrophy

Lower connectors can be either **bars** or **plates**—polymethylmethacrylate is too weak to be used as a bar so you are stuck with plates. Metal can, of course be used as either a bar or plate.

ONE THING YOU MUST KEEP IN MIND IS THAT YOU CANNOT STRENGTHEN THE LOWER DENTURE WITH A POSTERIOR BAR, IT WOULD LEAD TO SPEECH DIFFICULTIES AND OTHER PROBLEMS WITH THE TONGUE!

Have a look at some examples of lower dentures (next page).

Here are four lingual connectors and one buccal connector: lingual bar, including sub-lingual bar (1), lingual plate (2), dental bar (3), lingual bar plus a minor connector (continuous clasp) (4), buccal bar (5)*.

* Not included at this point is the buccal bar which should be self explanatory and should lie not less than 3 mm below the labial gingival margins (see p. 39).

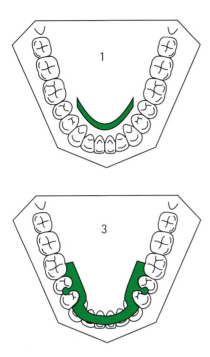

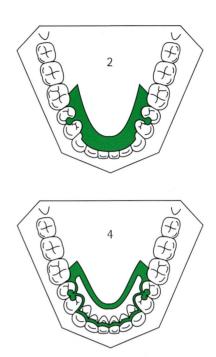

We will take these one by one, once you have had a look at them.

Lingual bar (1)

The lingual bar is either cast or wrought (the latter not recommended due to its poor fit). The bar must clear the gingival margins by at least 3 mm. The bar itself is normally about 3.5 mm at the greatest diameter and must be clear of the reflected sulcus. This is shown as a tooth supported and tooth and tissue supported version.

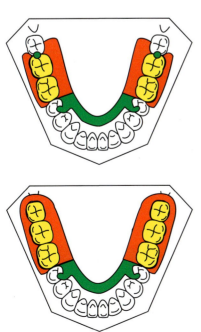

The bar may be oval (not good) or pear-shaped in section. The pear-shape is better tolerated by the tongue and reduces food trapping.

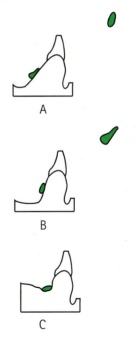

A sloping lingual contour (A) is satisfactory for a tooth supported denture, where there is no downward movement of the denture. Any downward movement of the bar would traumatize the underlying tissue, as would be the case if the saddles were tissue supported, therefore not recommended if there are no occlusal rests.

With an upright contour (B), vertical movement causes no damage (better).

If there is insufficient depth of sulcus to clear the gingival margins properly, a sub-lingual bar (C) can lie at the functional reflection of the lingual sulcus and not interfere with tongue movement.

Lingual plate (2)

The lingual plate is well tolerated, presenting a smooth surface to the tongue and is largely self-cleansing on the lingual surface.

The fact that it rests on the teeth means that it will act as an indirect retainer (Chapter 1.8) for free-end saddles (provided there are clasps in position, of course).

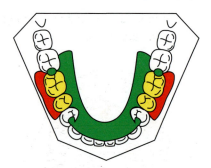

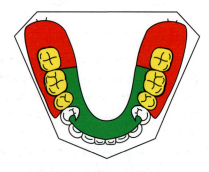

In the lower illustration, backward movement cannot take place as the denture base engages the mesial embrasures of the premolars and there are also occlusal rests.

On the down side, all the gingival tissues are covered, leading to loss of natural friction and stagnation. Oral hygiene must be meticulous.

Note that if only the anterior six teeth are standing, on loading the denture the plate can slide backward and downward and act as a 'gum stripper' unless there are rest seats on the canines and the denture base fitted into the lateral/canine lingual embrasures.

Dental bar (3)

The dental bar is rather like a shortened lingual plate. It lies on the teeth so avoiding gingival damage.

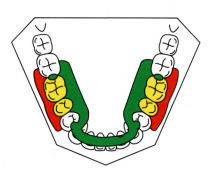

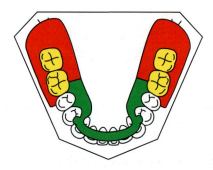

In cases of free-end saddles, indirect retention for the saddles is provided in conjunction with clasps (not shown) on the premolars. Downward and backward movements are prevented by the occlusal rests and the canine/premolar embrasures respectively.

Unfortunately, due to the reduced height available on the lingual sides of the teeth, the bar must be considerably thicker than a plate and therefore bulkier. This added bulk allows debris to collect and some patients do not tolerate well the intrusion into the area used by the tip of the tongue in rest and particularly in speech.

Lingual bar with minor connector (4)

You probably realize, given the comments on the last two connectors, that with free-end saddles the lingual bar can dig into the soft tissues if the rear of the saddles are lifted while chewing sticky foods. To counter this we can incorporate an indirect retainer (more of which later) such as a 'continuous clasp' as an accessory connector.

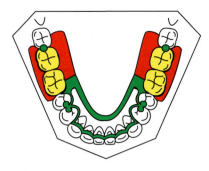

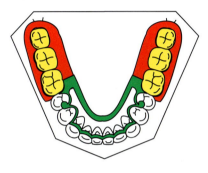

The extension will hold the posterior part of the denture in place by acting with clasps placed on the premolars (not shown).

The advantage of this design is that the gingival margins are kept clear, avoiding trauma and stagnation while improving the stability of the denture. On the other hand debris can collect on the teeth underneath and patients can find the extra part irritating.

Where there are free-end saddles, rests, clasps and the denture base must be designed to avoid backward movement, if not, the trauma to the soft tissues will be damaging.

Buccal bar (5)

This connector may be used when the lower anterior teeth or premolars are inclined lingually and the denture cannot be inserted because of the large lingual undercuts.

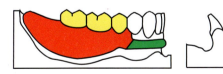

This applies mostly where there is a tooth or teeth instanding in the premolar region, so much so that the width between the occlusal surfaces of the contralateral teeth is much less than the width at the level of the gingival margins.

The buccal bar lies on the mucosa on the outside of the alveolus, and the denture must be stable to avoid trauma to the soft tissues.

Patient tolerance is not great and there is a tendency towards food stagnation about the bar, because it must be bulky enough to resist distortion in function and by the patient.

Every denture

Designed by its namesake to reduce damage to the remaining teeth as far as possible.

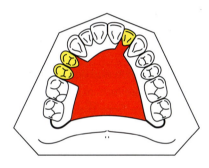

There is only point contact between the pontics and the standing teeth. The major retentive force is by a friction or 'jam' fit into place. This is the reason for the 1 mm wires on the distal surfaces of the molars. These are **not** clasps and only lie **on** the survey line and are to stop any backward drift of the posterior teeth which could compromise the friction fit of the denture. Major disadvantages are the loads which can be applied to the small tissue supported saddles and the narrowness of the connectors in these areas which can predispose to fracture of the denture base.

Spoon dentures

The spoon denture is popular for the replacement of one or two anterior teeth or as a temporary measure before the provision of a fixed appliance.

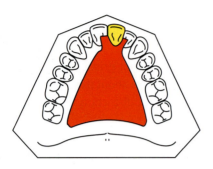

The gingival tissues are kept free, but do notice that the denture base has been extended to cover the cingula of the adjacent teeth. This coverage is vital to prevent excessive loading of the tissues below the artificial tooth and stripping of the gum around the abutments (the saddle is now effectively tooth supported).

Retention is by adhesion and cohesion and helped by a shallow 'dam line' (sometimes called a 'pin dam') around the periphery. Pressure from the tongue also holds the palate of the denture in place during incision, when the denture tends to tilt. Backward movement is prevented by the addition of a labial flange.

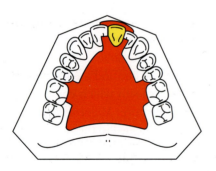

The lateral extensions shown in this figure add considerably to stability (taken above the survey line to avoid gingival damage) and clasps may be added to the molars.

These small dentures should be radio-opaque in case of displacement or fracture and subsequent loss by ingestion or inhalation. As commercial radio-opaque polymethylmethacrylate denture base material is not widely available, it is wise to insert some radio-opaque material into the denture during packing at the time of processing. This might be in the form of a little stainless steel wire or gauze.

Pause and reflect

By now you should have realized that we have been talking about the means to an end.

Connectors can be made in all shapes and sizes provided that you always remember that during the restoration of form and function which, after all, is the whole object, you avoid damage to any tissues either by action, such as gum stripping, or inaction such as excessive tissue coverage leading to stagnation.

We have been talking about rigid connectors, as stated in the beginning. There are, of course, other types of connectors such as those which are flexible or manufactured as precision devices to be included in the denture base (see Section 3).

Note: Never, ever design a unilateral denture that does not lock into position. Being small there is danger of inhalation or swallowing.

A comparison between cobalt chromium and acrylic resin as a denture base material

Cobalt chromium based dentures	Acrylic resin based dentures
Saddles and denture teeth have to be attached to the denture base	Saddles and denture teeth form part of the denture base
Stronger in thin section and therefore can be less bulky. High flexural strength	Need adequate thickness of material to ensure that it will not be vulnerable to fracture and therefore the prosthesis may become more bulky. Material is vulnerable to failure in flexion
High abrasion resistance	More vulnerable to abrasion
Method of construction more complex. Casting procedure involves the production of an investment model. Additional laboratory stage required to add the acrylic saddles and denture teeth. Potential for a greater casting shrinkage with certain designs	One stage procedure to construct the denture base incorporating the saddles and denture teeth. Polymerization contraction can be minimized in the processing of the resin
Can achieve tooth support by occlusal rests which form part of the framework	Tooth support not easily achievable with the resin itself. Although it is possible to embed cobalt chromium occlusal rests into it, this can be technically challenging
High thermal conductivity	Acts as a thermal insulator
Can minimize coverage of gingival margins for maxillary and mandibular dentures with favourable design features	Can minimize coverage of gingival margins with some maxillary dentures but due to limitations in strength, this is not normally achievable for mandibular dentures
Radio-opaque	Not normally radio-opaque without the incorporation of an additive or customized insert
More limited scope to make additions to the denture if further teeth are lost, particularly if they are not adjacent to a saddle	Generally simple procedure to make additions to the denture if further teeth are lost
Difficult to repair if a component fractures e.g. an isolated clasp not adjacent to a saddle	Often fractured components are simple to repair e.g. a clasp can be replaced easily

Conclusions

In this chapter we have described the types of connector available to join together saddles, rests, and clasps to create a safe, sufficiently strong and rigid partial denture base. Advantages and disadvantages of the designs have been identified.

Some points to remember

Whenever possible, choose a connector which:

- is as unobtrusive as possible—minimum bulk and tissue coverage, consistent with strength
- avoids coverage of gingival margins wherever possible

1.7 Retention

A removable partial denture must be held firmly in place. This is usually arranged by clasps, or part of the denture base, engaging hard tissue undercuts. The position and action of retainers must not damage any tissues. Special attachments are not considered in this chapter.

DESIGN SEQUENCE

teeth to replace
support
connectors
retention
refine

Before you start this chapter we expect you to be familiar with the chapter on surveying (Chapter 1.4).

The usual way of retaining partial dentures is by means of metal clasps. Direct retention is gained through a clasp which engages an undercut on a tooth and, through its resistance to removal from the undercut, holds that part of the denture in place.

The degree of resistance to removal of a clasp depends on three principal features:

- the flexibility of the arm (type of metal and whether wrought or cast)
- the length and cross-section of the arm
- the depth of the undercut engaged

Clasps are divided into two main types:

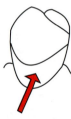

Occlusally approaching clasps are those which enter the undercut from the occlusal area of the tooth (upper diagram) and **gingivally approaching clasps** which enter the undercut by crossing the gingival margin.

Of the two, gingivally approaching clasps are the more efficient due to the 'trip action' when removal is attempted. Let us explain this action.

The '**trip action**' of gingivally approaching clasps is best explained by analogy. If you push a stick along the ground in front of you and it meets an obstruction, it will tend to dig in and be hard to move.

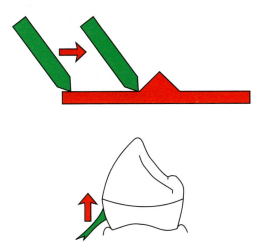

This is exactly what happens when you try to remove a gingivally approaching clasp from a tooth. The tip of the clasp is angled against the enamel in the undercut below the survey line and any attempt to remove it will make it try to dig in. This is called the '**trip**' action of the clasp.

Compare this to the action of an occlusally approaching clasp, using the same analogy, if you trail a stick along the ground behind you, it will just bump over any obstruction without difficulty.

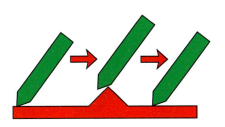

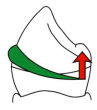

This is just what happens when an occlusally approaching clasp is pulled off a tooth. The tip of the clasp is dragged from the undercut and slides over the survey line. There is no '**trip**' action to enhance its retention.

Never forget that the **point of action of a clasp is at the tip** no matter where it arises from the denture base or how it gets into the undercut.

For the sake of simplicity in this chapter, we will only consider retention of a denture in the path of displacement, that is, a path at right angles to the occlusal plane.

Have a look at a few of the undercuts you may have to engage. You have already seen some common survey lines, similar to these, showing the greatest diameter of a tooth. Remember that above the survey line is the non-undercut area of the tooth, and below is the undercut area where we look for retention.

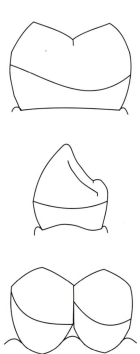

The undercut areas shown are quite good, in that there is plenty of room to place the tip of the clasp and they are easily approached occlusally or gingivally. However the size and shape of undercuts vary.

The type of clasp depends on the amount of undercut area available and whether there is enough of the undercut in the horizontal plane for the clasp to resist removal.

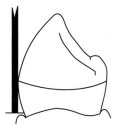

Standard crown

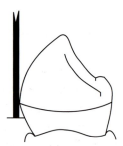

Bulbous crown

These illustrations show the same undercut gauge indicating the same horizontal undercut on teeth with differing buccal contours. The depth of the horizontal undercut engaged will depend on the resilience of the clasp arm.

So there are two major factors to consider, the **magnitude** of the undercuts in the **vertical plane** and the **horizontal plane**.

Here are three other examples of ways of entering undercuts.

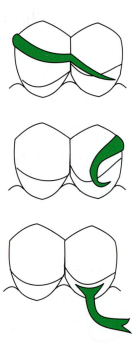

An occlusally approaching '**extended arm**', to engage an undercut where a nearer one is not satisfactory, is not often used nowadays unless the tooth adjacent to the saddle is crowned and has little undercut. Where teeth are not bulbous, composite resin can easily be added to enamel to provide an undercut (see later).

An occlusally approaching '**recurved arm**', to pick up an area next to a saddle, allows the arm to be long enough for flexibility.

A **gingivally approaching clasp** attached to a small shallow area provides good retention (trip action) and is hardly visible. Three more examples follow:

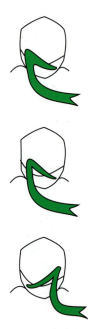

Gingivally approaching clasps are sometimes referred to as **roach clasps**.

> Some of these are given fancy names, such as **T, U, L, I** and **C**, these descriptions are just a shorthand for the shape of the retentive part of the arm.

Of course there are times, with very low survey lines, when the only useful retentive area is in the interdental embrasure. In these cases a ball-ended or arrowhead clasp can tuck into the gingival part of the interdental embrasure (occlusally approaching arms are usually wrought to give sufficient flexibility).

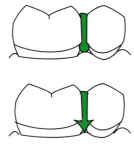

If the arm approaches from the gingival area, it can be made long enough to be of cast metal instead of wrought.

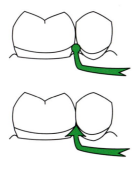

Should there be no undercut at all, then create one using one of these methods:

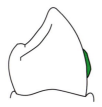

Added composite

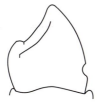

Depression in enamel

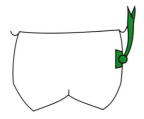

Inlay with depression or groove

- **Recontour** part of the tooth with composite resin—preferred method
- **Grind a depression** in the enamel (treat with fluoride) —preferably avoided
- **Fit an inlay** with a dimple or groove on the surface for a ball or ordinary arm to engage—useful if an inlay is considered due to caries or abrasion/erosion

Composite resin addition is the most common procedure, as it is reliable and the least destructive to tooth substance.

We have looked at the basic clasp types, action and placing. You should remember that no part of a partial denture design is isolated, there is an inter-relation with other aspects such as surveying, indirect retention, design, and manufacture of the clasp itself and so forth.

Many particular forms or shapes of clasp are given rather confusing or peculiar names. Do not bother overly with these, **just work out the best way to get into the undercut keeping in mind the properties of the material and that the point of action is at the tip.**

Next we must consider **reciprocal action** and **bracing**.

As the tip of a clasp passes into, or resists removal from, an undercut it exerts a sideways force on a tooth. You well know that the periodontal ligament can be damaged by this action, so such forces must be counteracted. There must be a balancing or **reciprocal action** to that of the clasp, provided by another part of the denture.

Reciprocal action (reciprocation)

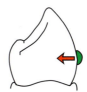

Unbalanced force

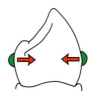

Balanced forces

The reciprocal action can be provided by another arm on the other side of the tooth; this arm lies on the survey line and is called the **reciprocal arm**. As it lies on the survey line it provides a balancing force but gives no retention (if the tip of this arm passed into an undercut area it would not only provide a reciprocal force but also add a retentive force).

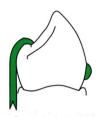

Vertical part of the denture base will be in contact during the whole period of insertion/removal

Reciprocal action (reciprocation) can also be provided by the denture base opposite the clasp, taken on to (and above if the design requires) the survey line.

A lone clasp arm places unacceptable lateral stresses on a tooth during insertion, removal and function, really an intermittent orthodontic appliance. *You should not design a clasp without reciprocal action.*

Bracing

Bracing is necessary to counteract lateral displacing forces applied to a denture. In this particular case bracing is supplied by clasps across the arch, the active arms buccally and the reciprocal arms palatally. When there are no clasps the denture base fitting against the teeth usually supplies sufficient bracing action.

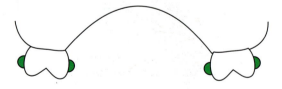

The reciprocal component, arm or denture base, also steadies the denture **against lateral movements** (as does any part of the active arm which lies **above** the survey line). This is called the **bracing action** and of course, is not confined to clasping areas; any part of the denture that resists applied lateral forces provides bracing.

Three definitions

- **Reciprocal action (reciprocation):** any component of a partial denture which prevents displacement of a tooth by a direct retainer.
- **Bracing action:** provided by a component of a partial denture which resists the action of lateral displacing forces on the denture.
- **Bracing:** resistance to horizontal components of force applied to the denture as a whole.

Guide planes

Guide planes are not clasps but are an important factor in retention and enhancing clasp action. The idea is to use or create paths of insertion and removal, which can improve and help in the retention and stability of a denture.

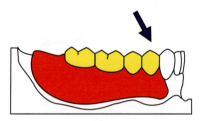

You can see a natural guide plane here, used to its best advantage. The denture is inserted along the line of the arrow and fits snugly into the distal undercut of the canine where it will resist vertical displacement.

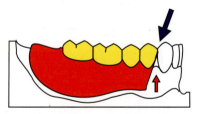

This next design is poor, badly surveyed and leaving a large food trapping gap (red arrow) between the denture and tooth. There is nothing to resist upward displacement of the denture.

Guide planes are prepared by adjusting the contours of teeth to allow a single straight path of insertion/removal of a saddle. That is to say if the opposing surfaces of the abutment teeth of a saddle are parallel, the fit will be more precise, there will be no dead space in undercuts and movement of the denture restricted to the exact path of insertion/removal.

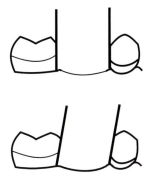

Teeth prepared with flat parallel planes
giving a precise paths of insertion/removal

Guide plane preparations should, of course, be confined to enamel.

Here you can see the preparation of a bulbous abutment tooth for a vertical path of insertion. The path of insertion will be precise and there will be greatly reduced dead space.

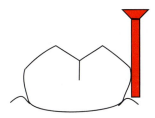

Analysing rod

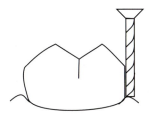

Bulbous part of the tooth removed

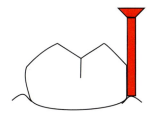

Guide plane established

Apart from making a precise line of insertion/removal, guide planes are sometimes used to make a flat area on a tooth surface for part of a denture which is providing reciprocal action (reciprocation) to a clasp arm. This flat area allows the reciprocal component to remain in contact with the tooth during the time the active arm is passing into, or out of, its undercut.

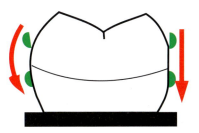

The RPI system (rest, plate, and I-bar), which we will be looking at next, uses guide planes.

You must always keep in mind that the removal of tooth tissue is not a procedure to be treated lightly and may even be considered by the patient to be mutilation. Make sure that any preparation is precise, smoothed, and treated with fluoride.

The RPI system

The **Rest**, **Plate**, and **I-bar** system is in common use and is normally placed on to the abutment tooth of a free-end saddle.

Guide planes are prepared, (mesiolingually) for the minor connector of the mesial rest and distally for the distal plate. The denture base contacting these planes provides reciprocal action for the retaining buccal I-bar and bracing for the denture.

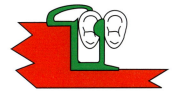

Occlusal view

Antero-posterior stability is provided by the rest and plate. Reciprocal action to the I-bar is from the rest connector.

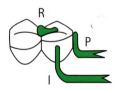

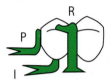

Buccal and lingual views

As this is a free-end saddle the denture sinks under load. The point of rotation is about the tip of the occlusal rest. The plate swings downwards and mesially and the I-bar swings further into the undercut.

The next diagram shows a multiple clasping system.

The essential parts of the clasping system are shown in **green** to make them easier to see.

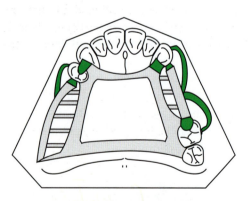

The tooth supported saddle cannot sink so its retention is not complex. The abutment of the tooth and tissue supported saddle is exactly as you saw in the last diagram. Guide planes are usually cut for the plates and the rest connectors (premolar and molar—not possible on the canine of course) so that the path of insertion is vertical (there might be some stability problems with this type of design but forget that for now).

Where to put clasps?

Thinking about retention for a partial denture is rather like wondering where to put the nails if you had to fix a wooden tile to the ceiling (to retain it).

Given four nails—use one at each corner—easy.

Excellent
Solidly attached

Given two nails, still an easy choice—common sense tells you that if you put a nail at opposite corners, or a nail half way along opposite sides, the tile would be held firmly in place.

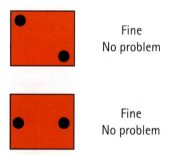

Fine
No problem

Fine
No problem

So far, no problem. But common sense also tells you that it would be rather stupid to put both the nails at one side, the weight of the tile would cause it to fall down at the opposite side. Look at the diagrams—you are supposed to be looking **up** at your handiwork.

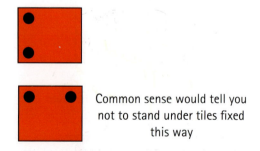

Common sense would tell you not to stand under tiles fixed this way

Check out the position of these clasps on a denture base.

Retention of the outlined denture base is good. Lines drawn through the **tips** of the clasps enclose almost the complete denture, so it will be held steady against displacing forces as shown in the next diagrams.

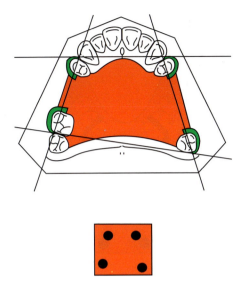

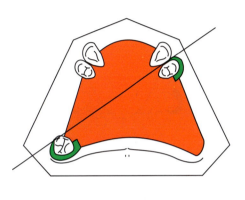

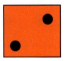

As you can see from the tile above, the side with only one nail is quite adequately held and there would be no danger of the tile falling.

Here is a denture with just two clasps, but as you can see the retention should be perfectly adequate if the clasps are strong enough.

Note: **The anterior clasp tips face mesially and the posterior clasp tips face distally, if the clasps had faced in the opposite direction, less of the denture base would have been included in the 'retentive' area.**

Comparing the denture to a nailed ceiling tile, the tile is held in place at all four corners and cannot fall.

With no upper right molars things are a little more difficult, however the triangle formed by joining the **tips** of the clasps includes the 'centre' of the denture.

The parts lying outside the triangle are **indirectly retained** (check your understanding of indirect retention later if you are not sure).

What story does the tile tell you? No real difficulty, there would be no danger from standing below this one.

On the other hand, the retention of this denture would not be adequate, as the posterior part presents such a long lever from the clasp axis that it would take very little force to dislodge it from the tissues.

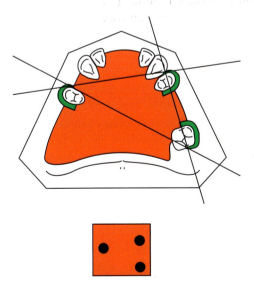

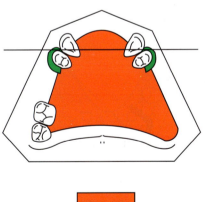

You would not be so happy standing beneath this one, would you? The unfixed side might be a bit too heavy for the nails to hold the tile up.

All that has been said about the upper dentures applies equally to displacement of lower dentures.

The next three illustrations are **lower dentures each having two clasps**. See how the effectiveness of the clasping differs.

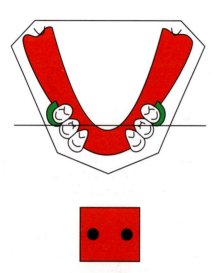

In the first case the clasping is reasonable to hold the denture in position. All the saddles are indirectly retained (see Chapter 1.8). The back of the denture cannot lift because the front cannot go down. Conversely the front cannot lift as the back cannot go down. The tile is looking good and is well held.

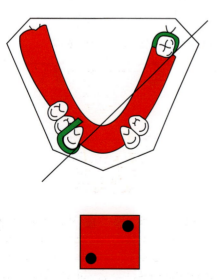

This denture should stay in place. Check out the tile.

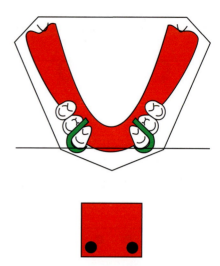

What of this then? What is there to hold the free-end saddles in place—nothing really. Look at the tile, the weight of the unfixed side is in danger of levering out the nails and the whole thing is liable to fall down.

Simplicity of design usually pays off—there is less to go wrong, it often makes oral hygiene easier and usually costs less to make.

Conclusions

You should now have some understanding of resistance to denture displacement during function, using undercut areas identified by surveying. Such undercuts can be employed for clasp placement and for selecting a path of insertion at variance with the likely displacing forces.

Some points to remember

- The first part of an occlusally approaching clasp provides bracing; the terminal third provides retention
- Gingivally approaching clasps can be more efficient than occlusally approaching clasps
- The point of action of a clasp is at the **tip** (no matter how it gets to that point)
- Beware of food traps e.g. unfilled undercuts or ball-ended embrasure clasps
- Do not remove tooth tissue unnecessarily (and without the patient's permission) for guide planes or rest seats

Adhesion, cohesion and surface tension help in the retention of upper dentures with palatal coverage, such as the 'spoon' and 'Every' dentures (as well as the patient's ability to develop effective tongue control)

Indirect retention

Indirect retention is a means of preventing the displacement of a saddle which is cantilevered out from the direct retainer(s), such as a free-end saddle or curved anterior saddle. A lever system must be created to keep the saddle in place.

DESIGN SEQUENCE

teeth to replace
support
connectors
retention
refine

Let us look at the forces involved in the retaining parts of partial dentures which cannot be held in place by direct means.

Indirect retention relates to saddles that cannot have a retainer at each end, or do not have the pontics in a straight line between the abutment teeth.

An example is a free-end saddle where there is only an abutment tooth at one end. Another example is an anterior saddle which is curved outside a straight line between the abutments.

It will be useful to be reminded of the Class III lever system, for it is the method by which indirect retention is effected. To help your memory of levers little diagrams have been added to many of the illustrations.

For a lower denture

Load (L)

or

Fulcrum (F) Effort (E)

F E

L

For an upper denture

Indirect retention is always a Class III lever system; it can never work at a mechanical advantage

Here is an everyday situation where a book or a tray is overhanging the edge of a table. In this instance let us suppose that it is a block of wood.

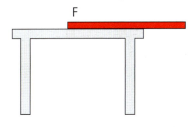

F

Look at the table and block from above

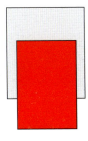

If you were to lift the block at the overhanging edge, then the opposite end would remain in contact with the table as the block hinged upwards, about its edge at **F**.

Apart from the weight of the block there is nothing to prevent this movement, is there?

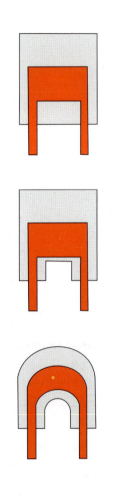

On the left you can see modifications have been made to the block and table. Whatever alterations are made, if the overhanging part is lifted, the other end will still lie on the table top and hinge about its edge.

Do you think that, with a little imagination, the third illustration on the left looks a bit like an outline partial denture (with free-end saddles) lying on an occlusal table?

You could stop the outer edge of the block being lifted by nailing the block to the table near to the table edge. Common sense tells you to put the nail near the edge, naturally you would not put the nail near the left hand edge of the block. Why?

Because you know that when you lifted the block the leverage would pull the nail out. This simple fact tells you how to make indirect retention work well.

Check the lever diagrams, as a Class III system the nearer E is to the lifting load L the better.

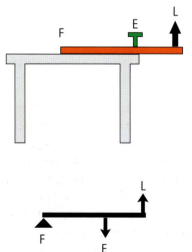

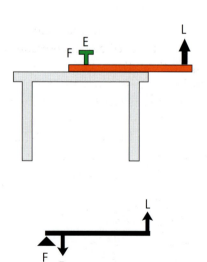

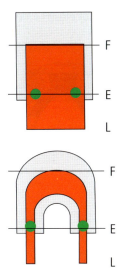

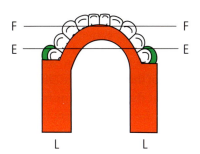

This rotation is not possible as the anterior part of the denture is lying on the teeth (occlusal table) and cannot move (forming the fulcrum), so lifting of the saddles will be resisted.

Looking at the next two illustrations (above), the same as the earlier examples but with added nails, you can see the addition of the nails and the lever system they have created will stop the overhanging part of the block from lifting. Therefore although the overhang cannot itself be directly fixed in position, it has been fixed in place indirectly by the table top acting as a fulcrum and the nails as the effort working together to prevent you lifting it.

Using a little imagination again, the lower illustration looks a bit like an outline partial denture lying on an occlusal table. With the teeth gripped at **E** the free-end saddles would be prevented from lifting (retained).

Applying our analogy of the red block representing a partial denture lying partly on the teeth and partly overhanging distally to replace the missing posterior teeth, it can be seen that if the posterior part were to be lifted, the denture would at first rotate about the axis **F-F** where it lies on the anterior teeth (as below). Then with further raising posteriorly the denture would just lift off the tissues altogether. This denture would not be retentive.

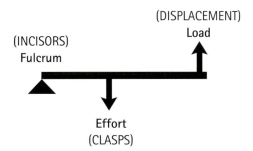

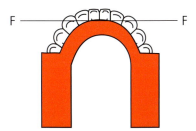

Look at the difference made by putting clasps on the premolars. If you try to lift the back of the denture, because of the grip of the clasps, it will *try* to rotate about the axis **E-E**.

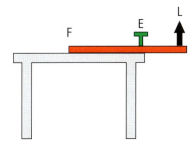

Here is the lever system which has been created. It is a **Class III** system because the **fulcrum** axis **must** be at the part which cannot move—the teeth at **F-F**. The (retaining) **effort** is at **E-E** where the clasps resist upward movement of the force trying to displace the saddles **(load)**.

The posterior part of the denture is now retained, not directly as there is no fixation at the back of the denture, but **indirectly** by the lever system.

Just to check, compare this to the table and block arrangement with which we started.

It is clear that a displacing force at **L** will be resisted by the nail at **E**, the fulcrum is at **F**.

Be clear as to why the fulcrum is at F. If the displacing force is strong enough the nail will be pulled out; therefore the nail **must** be the Effort (retainer). The part against the table cannot move, so it has to be the Fulcrum.

The saddles are *indirectly retained* by the standing teeth through the Class III lever system

Note: Did you realize that the jaw works as a Class III lever—the *L*oad is at the incisors, the *E*ffort at the elevators and the *F*ulcrum at the joint? Just as well our molars are further back than the incisors where the muscles can be more effective.

Now that the principle has been established, let us look more closely at partial denture design.

Partial dentures do not normally lie **on** the teeth; tooth support is usually derived through occlusal rests arising from the denture base or modifying part of the denture base to act as a rest. Therefore the denture is only supported by the teeth where the design dictates. This illustration outlines a denture utilizing no tooth support at all. It is also non-retentive.

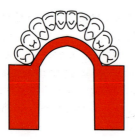

You can see from the next diagram that

Clasps alone will allow a rotation about the clasp tips where the tooth is gripped.

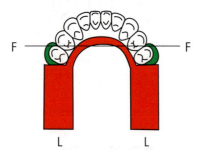

Because there is no part of the denture lying on the teeth anterior to the clasps, there is nothing to prevent the anterior part of the denture moving down towards the floor of the mouth. There is no proper lever system. There is a load and a fulcrum but no effort, so there is nothing to prevent the posterior part of the denture from lifting.

You have just seen that **clasps alone** only hold one part of the denture steady.

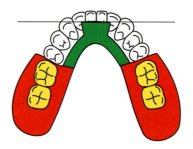

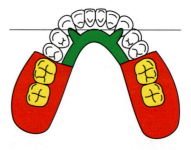

Looking at these two diagrams, it is clear that **rests alone** do nothing to retain the denture base, the whole thing can just be lifted off. If the posterior end only were lifted the denture would hinge up on the rests which are lying passively on the teeth, there is nothing to hold them, or the denture, in place.

So you can see that indirect retention of a saddle cannot be achieved by clasps or rests acting on their own.

Indirect retention can only be achieved through a combination of clasps and rests to form a lever system to retain the free part of the denture.

So let us now **combine the actions of the clasps and rests** we have been discussing into a working unit which will retain the free-end saddles.

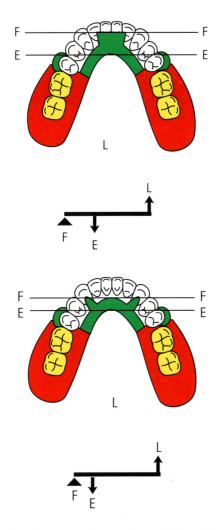

Here, then, is a complete system which will retain the free-end saddles.

Observe, however, the relationship of clasps to fulcra.

You know that changing the lengths of the lever arms alters the efficiency of the system, and this will alter the degree of indirect retention possible.

The fulcrum is at **F-F**, so when the lever arm **FE** is working against the arm **FL**, which is the part to be stopped from moving (retained), the greater the distance between the rests and the tips of the clasps the better, as it lengthens the retaining lever.

This means that the upper diagram is the more efficient design as the retaining lever (**FE**) is the longer.

As the retaining ability of the clasps is limited to the force required to drag them off the teeth, the upper diagram is still the design of choice.

How about this for a design?
Look at the lengths of the levers.

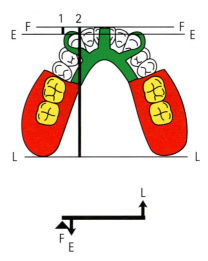

The retaining lever (**1**) is so short that it would be useless against the leverage of the displacing force (**2**), unless the clasp was enormously strong—so strong that it would apply an extracting force on to the tooth with relatively little displacing force applied to the saddle.

The retaining lever must be as long as possible (Fulcrum to Effort).

Consider the next design:

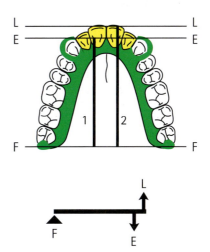

This shows a design for missing upper incisors: this is mechanically very good. Look and see where the fulcrum is.

The fulcrum axis is through the posterior rests at **F-F** and any displacing force applied at the incisors to remove the denture (on the lever arm between **L** and **F** (**2**) is resisted by the lever arm between **E** and **F** (**1**) which is almost the same length.

Note: **We are only concerned here with theory, not aesthetics or the amount of tissue coverage. These are factors which may cause modification of the design at a later stage.**

For instance, in the last example, the tips of the clasps may have to be placed further back for aesthetic reasons, which would reduce the retaining efficiency.

By now you should be able to draw up different designs; indirect retention is quite simple if you look at it from the point of view of a simple lever system.

Let us suggest a definition: an *indirect retainer* is a **supporting** element on the other side of a line joining the tip(s) of the **retaining** element(s).

Note: Beware of any definitions you might see which refer to a line joining the clasps as the *Fulcrum*. You have seen that this is *not* correct, as the clasps can be levered out of position, and is quite misleading as far as the effectiveness of the retention is concerned. This assumption makes the system appear to be a Class I lever which it certainly is not.

It has probably occurred to you that designs are not always symmetrical, as you can see from this example:

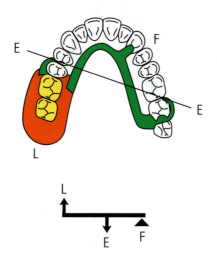

The lever principle still holds good, as the saddle at (L) cannot lift, can it?

No, the displacing force is applied to the lever **LF** and is resisted by the lever **EF** (E being the distance from **F** to the line **E-E**, of course).

All you have to do is work out the best lever system for each design when part of the denture is cantilevered out from areas which can be directly retained.

One other thing before we finish. The denture base itself can be used to gain indirect retention.

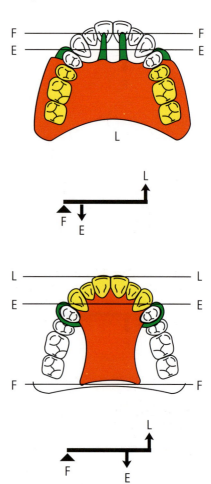

In both cases the denture base has been extended beyond a line joining the tips of the clasps.

In the upper diagram '**Cummer arms**' have been incorporated to form cingulum rests on the central incisors; these will form the indirect retainers to stop the back of the denture falling. Not very efficient in this case, but nonetheless helpful. In the example illustrated, there is potential for food stagnation around the closely placed Cummer arms. Extension of the acrylic base around the anterior teeth would also provide indirect retention but covering the gingival margins could be considered a disadvantage.

The last diagram shows a backward extension of the denture base, beyond a line connecting the tips of the clasps, which will act as an indirect retainer to stop the front of the denture falling. A very considerable help in this case.

A further point to keep in mind.

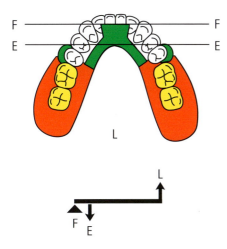

You have seen this diagram before, but looking at it again can you see how the indirect retention of the saddles could be improved?

Just think *where* each force is applied.

Answer:

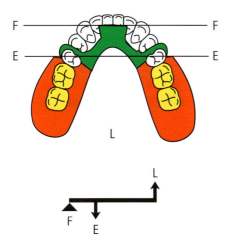

By changing the direction of the clasps, the rest/clasp lever is lengthened by moving the tips of the clasps (points of action) further away from the fulcrum (rest).

Here is a tissue supported denture.

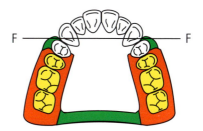

There is minimum tissue coverage and the gingival margins of the standing teeth are free from cover. The posterior palatal bar is well back keeping the palate free and avoiding tongue action; reciprocal action is provided by the denture base.

All very laudable, apart from the fact that the denture will not stay up. It will rotate about the tips of the direct retainers (clasps) and will be absolutely useless. *Think your designs through!*

> Do not be persuaded that indirect retention is a Class II, or even a Class I lever system. This presupposes that the clasp(s) is the fulcrum. This is not the case, as the fulcrum is on the teeth (which do not move) and the effort is the tip of the clasp(s) (which can move).
>
> The principle and application is simple once understood.

Conclusions

Indirect retention is often considered to be a 'difficult' concept. In this chapter we have tried to explain it, because it is an essential feature of many dentures especially when free-end saddles are required, as in Kennedy class I and II designs.

> **Some points to remember**
>
> Be sure that you have grasped the following:
>
> - the displacing **load** (sticky food) is applied to, for example, a free-end saddle as the mouth opens
> - the prosthesis will try to displace by rotation about the **fulcrum** created by the most distant supporting component of the denture from the saddle, perhaps a cingulum rest in the case of the free-end saddle(s)
> - resistance to movement, the **effort**, will be provided by the clasp(s) placed as far away from the fulcrum as possible

Indirect or cantilevered support

Indirect support provides support for a saddle which is cantilevered out beyond the area of available tooth support. The action is one of a Class I lever system and can therefore be very effective or very poor, depending on how the load, effort, and fulcrum are distributed.

You do not come across this term very often, but all the same it can be a vital factor in partial denture design whether you realize it or not.

We prefer the term **indirect support** as in its way it mirrors indirect retention. The former resists movement of a saddle towards the tissues (giving support) and the latter resists movement away from the tissues (giving retention).

Before beginning it would be as well to check again the existing principles of levers so that we know exactly what we are talking about.

We are going to look at this system of support with care, because in some cases it can be vital to the stability of a denture and in others may cause considerable damage to the teeth. It can easily be introduced inadvertently when retention is being considered. It all revolves around the **Class I** lever system.

Class 1 lever system

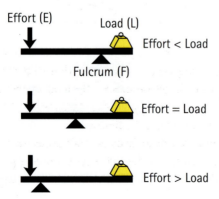

The concept is straightforward and, as with indirect retention, depends on a simple lever system as the saddle requiring tooth support is outside the area of the standing teeth. It is rather like a springboard sticking out from the side of a swimming pool. The side of the pool represents the solid standing teeth which provide support for the part overhanging the water which represents the soft compressible tissues.

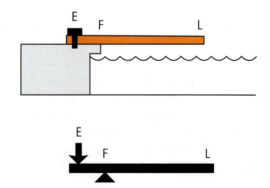

The Effort (fixing bolts) must be more than able to support the weight of a diver bouncing on the other end. In this case the system is working at a considerable **mechanical disadvantage**.

The saddles are often tissue supported, with rests anteriorly to pass some of the load to the teeth. There is a degree of choice, we will come back to this type of case later; so we will begin with a straightforward problem.

Let us look at the case of replacing four upper incisors where stability is vital. This saddle, if tooth supported, must be stable and the load should be carried by the canines. There should be no movement of the denture base. On the other hand a tissue supported denture could move, as it lies on resilient soft tissues, and could give the patient a sense of insecurity.

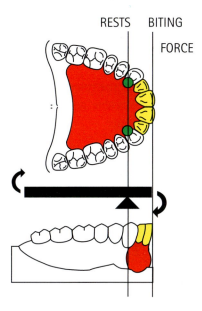

There is one big problem with the tooth supported idea and that is the arch of the anterior teeth. The incisal edges will normally be labial to a straight line joining the supporting points (cingula of the canines) and the saddle will lie on compressible soft tissue. So when the patient bites on the incisors the most anterior part would compress the soft tissues by swinging on an arc from the cingula of the uncompressible canines. This denture would be quite unsatisfactory, so a design must be developed to solve the problem.

Let us go back to the springboard analogy again.

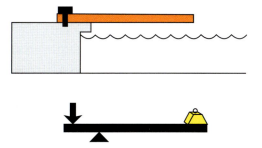

You would be quite happy (as a swimmer) to stand at the end of a springboard, wouldn't you? You can however imagine the problem that someone preparing to dive from the board would have if the bolts were not strong enough to balance the diver's weight.

You can apply this analogy to the tooth supported anterior saddle. The denture will only be stable if it is not allowed to tip towards the tissues, so the denture base must be secure enough not to move when the incisors bite through a bolus. In other words, the only way to stop the denture (springboard) from tilting is to make sure that rotation cannot take place about the rests (edge of the pool).

It is essential that the bolts securing the springboard are both strong enough and firmly fixed enough to withstand the fattest person jumping up and down at the far end of the board.

Similarly the denture base must be stopped from rotating about the rests, so the anterior saddle will be prevented from sinking on to the soft tissues underneath it.

Look at the mechanics of this.

If the back of the denture is fixed in position by clasps then rotation about the rests cannot take place. Notice the shift in position of the fulcrum, compared to the springboard, as the 'overhang' is much less. This **Class I** system works at a **mechanical advantage**.

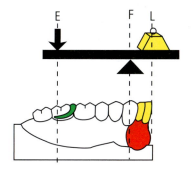

The **Class I** lever system now created means that the biting forces on the anterior teeth are balanced by the retaining forces of the clasps. **No** load is applied to the tissues under the saddle, as the clasps prevent the saddle from moving towards the tissues.

Therefore, as the anterior part of the denture cannot be easily moved towards the soft tissues (unless the clasps are displaced), the denture will be more stable in function.

In a **Class I** lever system it is obvious to the user that the greater distance the Effort is from the Fulcrum the better (less effort needed to lever up the lid of a tin by using a long screwdriver). Likewise the nearer the Fulcrum to the Load the greater the load that can be moved or balanced (same reasoning).

This explanation is fine in everyday terms, but with partial dentures we are looking at the **same** things from a different viewpoint, that is to say: the greater the distance the clasps (effort) are from the rests (fulcrum) *the less is the force required to balance the biting load (load)*.

Likewise the nearer the rests (fulcrum) to the incisors (load) *the greater the biting force can be without displacing the denture*.

In other words *the greater the distance between the clasps and the rests the better* (effort to fulcrum distance). *The nearer the rests to the incisors the better* (load to fulcrum distance).

It is essential that you have fully understood these facts. Now for some examples.

Here are three different designs for the same case:

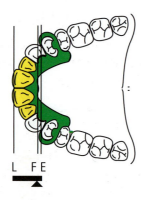

The first is quite neat, but you can see that the leverage is such that even a light biting force is liable to pull the clasps off the teeth—not such a good idea.

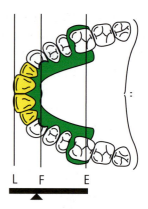

This is quite different, the retentive force of the clasps is working at a considerable advantage over the load. Excellent—a stable denture.

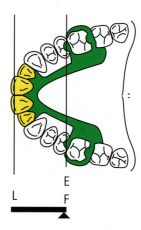

In this design the saddle is **not tooth supported** as we would prefer, it is virtually **tissue supported**. On loading, the denture would swivel about the premolar rests with the clasps hardly having any effect (apart from essential retention that is, but we are not looking at that just now).

So *do not confuse cantilevered support with retention*.

Some observations

You may think that the case of the upper anterior saddle has had a lot of attention. This may be true, but it is a common condition and one where a poorly designed tooth supported denture can do a lot of damage if rocking is not prevented during function. Further, the patient is aware if there is movement of the denture. This is the last thing you want, as patients should feel that the prosthesis is a part of themselves. Movement is a constant reminder of the denture and a worry that it might be noticed by others.

We noted that you should not confuse support with retention. Remember that all stages of design are inter-related, so **whenever** you work with rests and clasps you must think of the effect of the lever systems you are creating.

As an instance, look again at the last design where the anterior teeth were not tooth supported.

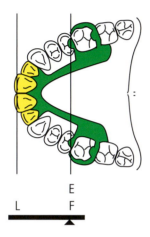

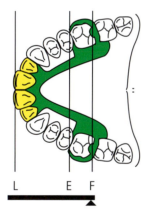

Suppose the canines were in very poor condition, so we decided to make the denture tissue supported. Removing the rests on the premolars will ensure that the denture will no longer rock about the rests but will just hinge a little about the part of the clasp that passes through the occlusal embrasure, this is so far from the saddle that it will not be noticeable. The denture is now virtually tissue supported and as stable as a tissue supported appliance can be, from the point of view of support.

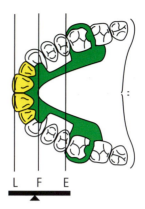

On the other hand, with sound teeth, move the rests (fulcrum) from the premolars to the canines and you have a good tooth supported design (almost identical to the stable design we considered earlier). The lever system would be further improved if the tips of the molar clasps pointed distally, as this would lengthen the lever for the effort, as in the earlier design.

It should be pretty clear to you now that the application of simple lever systems to partial denture design is vital.

You might now like to reflect upon just how important cantilevered support is in the design of tooth supported anterior saddles.

Look at a less than satisfactory scene

Lever systems such as we have been discussing can be introduced into designs unthinkingly with results that can cause considerable damage.

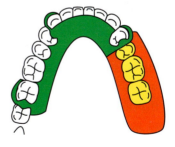

Look at this design—it looks reasonable doesn't it? (You know something must be wrong or the question would not have been asked.)

Have a good look at it. What do you find?

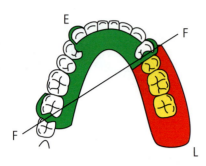

This is a common enough design but you have no doubt realized that the fulcrum axis is about the most distal rests (of course), and biting on the free-end saddle would cause compression of the underlying tissues.

As the saddle sinks the denture will rotate about the fulcrum, and the clasp on the canine will be displaced upwards. This denture is a 'rocker'. You can imagine the damage done to the canine by the continued movement of the clasp on the enamel. You could, of course, try and make the clasp so strong *that it would not move*—and end up with a mobile tooth because of the extracting leverage applied by the denture.

What can be done? Try some modifications.

How about this?

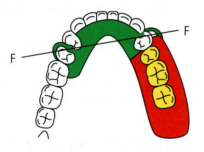

- By moving the rests forward the amount of rock is greatly reduced.
- Removing the canine clasp stops the abrasion of that tooth. What good did that clasp do anyway? (The denture is indirectly retained as it is.)
- The **indirect retention** is reduced because although the right premolar clasp is untouched, the mesial-facing molar clasp on the left has been replaced by a distal-facing clasp on the premolar (so the point of action has been moved a bit further forward). The indirect retainer (lingual plate) is unaffected.

The result is a more stable denture which hardly moves in function and tooth damage is avoided.

Finally it should be emphasized that when you design a partial denture, if there is a saddle or saddles which cannot be directly supported or retained, think through the effect on the whole denture of every rest and clasp you add.

There is no exact design to suit every case which presents, but if you understand the basic physics involved in design, you cannot go far wrong. It is not surprising therefore, that three different clinicians will produce three different designs for the same case. The dentures however should all be satisfactory but allowing for some 'give and take', for example sacrificing a little retention for better aesthetics, or additional gingival margin coverage to achieve better indirect retention or support.

Conclusions

The key to understanding the problem of indirect support is the 'springboard' analogy with which the chapter began. **Load** applied to the end of the springboard (free-end saddle, or long anterior saddle) will only be supported by the underlying tissue, with the risk of the denture rocking about rests on the abutment teeth acting as the **fulcrum**. Some resistance (**effort**) to this rock (and an aid to support) may be achieved by clasp placement as far away from the fulcrum as possible. However this may disadvantage the clasped tooth unless it is large and healthy. Furthermore there is always the possibility that if the denture does rock, the consequent movement of the clasp might abrade that tooth.

> **Some points to remember**
>
> There may be no single 'correct' solution to support, but the following may be helpful:
>
> - reduce the **load** by saddle design (narrow the occlusal table, omit the last molar for posterior saddles; compromise on anterior tooth position to reduce the cantilever effect)
> - only seek indirect support by clasping sound, healthy teeth

Refining the design

When a denture design is complete, it is time to step back and look at it anew. Every step might have been followed to the best advantage but is the final denture really satisfactory from the view of aesthetics, interplay of the elements of indirect retention and indirect support, and freedom from interferences with the tongue and other tissues? Review the complete design and make any necessary adjustments.

DESIGN SEQUENCE

teeth to replace
support
connectors
retention
refine

Once you have built up a denture design, step by step, it is time to stand back and look at the overall product.

There follows a number of points to be considered before a design is finalized. Some may cause you to modify your final design.

Tooth supported prostheses

- Have all the necessary teeth been replaced?
- Is the load the denture will bear distributed fairly and safely to the standing teeth?
- Are the connectors unobtrusive and do they minimize stagnation areas, only crossing the gingival margins in self-cleansing areas?
- Is the denture sufficiently large so that it cannot be swallowed or inhaled?
- Is retention sufficient and the retainers unobtrusive?

Remember that:

- thinner broader connectors, such as palatal bars are more acceptable than those which are narrow and thick. The same applies to clasp arms and occlusal rests

- clasps may not be acceptable to the patient if they are visible. Anterior clasps especially should be inconspicuous
- labial flanges should replace the interdental papilla at each end of the saddle and be extended over half the adjacent tooth to blend with the surrounding tissues (provided that the path of insertion allows this)
- there must be no occlusal interferences from rests or clasp connectors
- where there is a deep overbite and no natural teeth to establish the vertical height, the vertical dimension must not be raised by the lower anterior teeth striking the upper denture behind the incisors

Tissue supported appliances

- Include the above but be sure that the greatest possible area of mucosa is covered and the occlusal area is reduced to a minimum to reduce the tissue loading.
- Are the gingival margins, particularly of teeth adjacent to a saddle, free from any 'gum stripping' action as the denture sinks in function?
- No part of a clasp should be close to a gingival margin otherwise sinkage of the denture, during function or with time, will cause gingival damage.
- Is the denture liable to cause damage to the remaining teeth and gingivae as the denture sinks due to tissue and bone remodelling over time?

- Ensure that no part of the denture base lies above a survey line where it will apply a lateral force to the tooth when the denture is loaded.
- Remember that almost any attempt to provide indirect retention will convert the denture to a tooth and tissue supported type as the indirect retainer, however distant from the saddle, will act as a tooth supporting element when the saddle is loaded.

Tooth and tissue supported appliances

In addition to the points raised in the previous paragraphs:

- check every rest to be sure it is providing the **support** for which it is intended, in other words that it is not on the lifting side of a fulcrum formed by a rest nearer the tooth and tissue supported saddle. This does not include rests provided for indirect retention
- further ensure that no part of the denture base is above the survey line between the saddle and nearest supporting rest as this will produce lateral thrusts when the saddle is loaded
- check that the rests (or parts of the denture base above the survey line) providing **indirect retention** are as far away from the saddle(s) (and clasps) as possible
- the position of all clasps must be examined to see that they are not placed where extracting or abrasive forces can be applied to the teeth as the tissue supported part of the denture sinks in function or with time
- check that as far as possible the gingival margins of the teeth adjacent to a saddle are protected from damage

Conclusions

Refining is an important step in the development of a design. You should assess what you have created so far; is the potential for benefit to the patient maximized, but the risk of damage minimized?

Some points to remember

Check everything!

- Does your initial decision about the teeth that need to be replaced still seem wise?
- Is the support provision adequate (it is possible to over provide)?
- Is the connector(s) you have chosen appropriate?
- Are there enough clasps?
- Will the indirect retention work?
- Can changes be made to improve oral hygiene?
- What needs to be done **before** recording working impressions, such as restorations, periodontal treatment, tooth preparation?
- Where there is a free-end saddle(s), be very sure that your placement of clasps for retentive purposes does not introduce unintended indirect support, which, if the clasp is not sufficiently retentive, will abrade the tooth as the denture rocks under load

Section 2

The patient and the denture

The objective of this section is to provide a basic introduction to the process of application of the principles of partial denture design to the individual patient, building on the fundamental concepts explored in Section 1.

A series of short chapters will develop the process, starting with the essential investigation of the patient—medical and dental history including any previous denture experience. On the basis of this, the advisability of whether to provide partial dentures or not can be assessed.

If a partial denture, or dentures, can be judged to be advantageous, then it is appropriate to proceed to actual design. Articulated and surveyed casts of the mouth are needed to provide a precise indication of the relationship of the upper and lower teeth. With the help of this record, a decision can be made on which missing teeth should be replaced, to improve appearance and maintain of function.

It is convenient to adopt the Kennedy classification (Chapter 1.3) to proceed to provisional design decisions, because the fundamental problems vary significantly between the classical types. Each class will be allocated its own short chapter, starting with the most straightforward (Kennedy class III) and progressing to the more difficult.

Patient histories and assessment

Find out as much as possible about the patient.

Medical history

A full medical history must be recorded.

There are several elements which have important implications for maintained dental health and for denture use in particular.

Oral hygiene depends on salivary function, adequate self care and professional assistance. Especially in older patients any or all of these may be doubtful. Some examples of such conditions are:

- drug-induced xerostomia (dry mouth)
- impaired manual dexterity
- uncertain motivation of self care
- limited mobility restricting continuing care

In addition there are some specific medical conditions which contraindicate or may result in denture-wearing difficulties.

- epilepsy (swallowing/inhalation/fracture)
- Sjögrens syndrome/radiotherapy
- neurological conditions such as Parkinson's disease

Dental history

A full and detailed dental history must be recorded.

The state of the residual dentition is a good initial indicator of the past oral care. There may have been tooth loss which then initiated an improvement in self care. There may be records of past professional care, to add to the assessment of existing periodontal and restorative conditions. Present and previous denture experience is also important, and may provide useful evidence for the design of replacement(s). A design may be repeated if it has proved successful, and if no damage can be observed. Conversely an unsuccessful denture, or one which has caused damage, indicates the need for a design reassessment.

Current dental state

It is not necessary to embark upon denture provision in isolation from other aspects of care. It may often be appropriate to attend to oral hygiene instruction, periodontal therapy, and tooth restoration or extraction as an integral part of treatment.

A thorough clinical examination and full assessment not only of the remaining teeth, but also of the mouth as a whole is essential, including any necessary radiographs. Apart from the factors outlined, others may include:

- temporomandibular joint mobility/function
- muscle function
- salivary gland secretions

Denture history

The denture history may well be reflected in the dental history ranging from indifference to acute awareness.

Four possibilities may present:

- an existing denture which has been successfully used, but about which the patient is now critical (perhaps due to recent changes in the dentition)
- a previous but unsuccessful denture
- a patient request for replacement of a missing tooth or teeth; there may be no previous denture and tooth loss may be recent
- examination identifies advantages for the patient by provision of a denture. The patient may express a preference for a fixed appliance (bridge or implant)

Previous dentures

Examination of previous partial dentures is extremely valuable, providing information for consideration. Sometimes such dentures will have been successful in the patient's view, but this does not necessarily mean that all is, or was, well—damage could still have been occurring.

Irrespective of the patient's view, the dentures must be evaluated, ideally using the same criteria as would be used to design a new prosthesis:

- Appropriate tooth replacement?
- Are the dentures supportive or destructive?
- Adequate support?
- Hygienic and tolerable connector(s)?
- Retention effective and well distributed?
- Should a tissue conditioner be added to tissue supported saddles to improve the state of the underlying mucosa before a new denture is made?

Unsuccessful dentures should always be examined, both in and out of the mouth. Can reasons for the failure be found, or can alternative strategies be produced to overcome the failure (which can be on only one aspect of function, for example, acceptable appearance, but lack of retention or comfort)?

Conclusions

You should be, as well as is possible, fully informed about your patient. You should also be able to make a judgement —perhaps subjective—of the type of patient, for instance, their attitude to self care.

There is much of relevance to be obtained by careful investigation of the patient's medical and dental background.

Some points to remember

Medical and dental history may exert major influences upon decisions regarding overall dental care, including provision of partial dentures.
Look for:

- medical conditions which may affect denture design and prognosis
- potential difficulties and motivation for self care
- dental treatment history and the possible need for restorative work prior to denture provision

Articulated study casts

Accurate, articulated study casts enable a detailed assessment of the occlusion and of the morphology of the remaining dentition.

Accurate decisions on denture type and design require study casts of the upper and lower jaws, reproducing all relevant structures—all the retained teeth, and the functional depth of the sulci (buccal, labial, and lingual). The casts must be articulated in a manner which precisely records the jaw relationship.

When there are enough natural teeth present, this articulation process may be simple: reproduction of the existing intercuspal relationship in the mouth can be checked against tooth contacts on the casts.

If fewer teeth remain, it will be necessary to use record blocks to transfer the residual intercuspal position from the mouth to the casts. In addition it will be necessary to check that the patient's chosen closed position is appropriate as the intercuspal position. For instance, a patient retaining only anterior teeth may habitually protrude the mandible. The most useful test for this possibility is to seek the most retruded position of the mandible by closure with the tongue tip held against the soft palate, and to compare this with the habitual position. A difference of more than 1 mm (horizontally) indicates a protrusion habit, in which case the retruded contact position should be recorded to restore the correct physiological occlusal position.

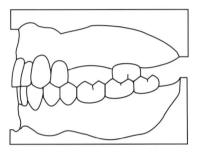

Normal

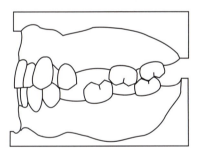

Drifting/overeruption

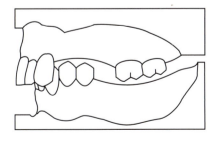

Overclosure/overeruption

Terminology reminder

Intercuspal position (ICP) = centric occlusion
Retruded contact position (RCP) = ligamentous position/
centric relation
Postural position = rest position
Freeway space = interocclusal space

On occasions, when few teeth remain, closure may go too far as there are no restrictions on how far the mandible can be elevated until the teeth contact the opposing soft tissues. Such overclosure should not normally be incorporated into a denture design. Instead the jaw relationship should be recorded so as to provide a free-way space between the relaxed (postural) position of the mandible and the intercuspal position. This is usually in the order of 2–4 mm, measured vertically with the head upright.

Cast surveying

The casts must be surveyed:

- first, with the occlusal plane horizontal, to show all the hard and soft tissue undercuts which lie in the path of displacement. The effective part of all retainers must lie in these undercuts if the denture is to remain seated during function

- second, with the cast tilted, to show the undercuts in the chosen path of insertion/removal. The effective part of the retainers must also lie within these undercuts to prevent movement of the denture in this path

- the second survey is usually necessary to avoid unsightly spaces between the denture and the natural teeth and gingival tissues

- should the chosen path of insertion/removal be the same as the path of displacement then, of course, a single survey is sufficient.

Revision of Chapter 1.4 is strongly recommended.

This completes the preparatory work, so it is now time to move on to the design of the individual denture.

Conclusions

Surveying is an essential process. If there are any doubts in your mind, please review Chapter 1.4.

Study casts, accurately articulated, are a vital component of treatment planning because it is essential to determine that there is sufficient space to locate the denture components without creating interferences in the occlusion.

Some points to remember

Remember that:

- study casts must be complete and accurate, deficiencies could render them worse than useless

- accurate articulation is essential to reproduce occlusal contacts

- record blocks may be needed to achieve correct articulation when few natural teeth remain

Which teeth to replace?
Design sequence

It is not always an advantage to replace all missing teeth. The question of whether to replace missing teeth is considered.

It is not always necessary or appropriate to replace all missing teeth. The importance of replacement could be said to diminish posteriorly, and on occasions it may be preferable to avoid denture provision altogether, but here are some guidelines:

- anterior tooth loss creates a major incentive for replacement
- natural teeth in one jaw, unopposed in the other, may possibly be at risk of gradual over-eruption especially in younger patients
- teeth on either side of an area of tooth loss may drift and tilt
- molar teeth at the distal end of a free-end saddle may usefully be omitted, unless an opposing natural tooth would be free to over-erupt

A decision on which teeth warrant inclusion on a partial denture leads to consideration of the basic classification of the partial denture(s) required:

Below is listed an intentional departure from the original numerical sequence of the Kennedy classification, for it is in this modified order that the next chapters will proceed.

Kennedy III: one or more bounded saddles

Kennedy II: one free-end saddle, possibly with one or more additional bounded saddles

Kennedy I: two free-end saddles, perhaps with additional bounded saddle(s)

Kennedy IV: a single anterior saddle (bounded)—technically defined as crossing the mid-line

Examination of the surveyed and articulated casts

Look for the following:

- undercuts on the teeth which dictate a suitable path of insertion for the denture (Chapter 1.4)
- undercuts on the teeth which could be used for clasp location (Chapter 1.7)
- undercuts which will interfere with insertion and removal of the denture. These may be on the teeth, or in the saddle areas of the soft tissues (Chapter 1.4)

It is then possible to embark upon the development of a design.

A drawn outline is an essential aid (see Appendix 1 for a suggested design proforma), together with coloured pencils, the usual colour code being:

- red—acrylic resin
- green—cast cobalt chromium
- yellow—gold (usually wrought wire clasps)
- blue—stainless steel (wrought wire clasps)

The following sequence of design is recommended:

- draw saddles
- add support components (rests)
- select connector(s)
- add retainers (clasps)
- consider the need for, and availability of, indirect retention

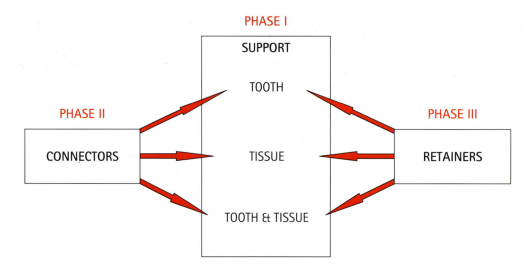

- consider the option of indirect support
- relate the provisional design to the opposing dentition (is there space for rests and clasps without occlusal interference?)
- look carefully at the oral hygiene implications (minimal gingival coverage and avoidance of food traps)

This is shown diagrammatically above.

Conclusions

A combination of history and articulated casts enables you to decide which (if any) missing teeth should be replaced by partial dentures. It is then possible to identify the Kennedy classification (Chapter 1.3). You may then proceed to the relevant chapter (Kennedy III, Chapter 2.4; Kennedy I and II, Chapter 2.5; Kennedy IV, Chapter 2.6).

Some points to remember

Key points are:

- in deciding which teeth to replace, weigh up the advantages and disadvantages for overall maintenance of oral health and function
- an overall course of treatment may include remedial restoration of some teeth and of periodontal health—it may also be necessary to prepare some teeth for the denture(s), for example, occlusal rest seats, guide planes

Designing for Kennedy class III dentures

Kennedy class III deals only with **bounded** saddles. **Remember** that 'modifications' account for any other bounded saddles present (see Chapter 1.3)

Saddle design

This is generally straightforward, although it is worthwhile to consider a fixed prosthesis (bridge) if the 'saddle' is short and the abutments periodontally sound.

Here are two examples:

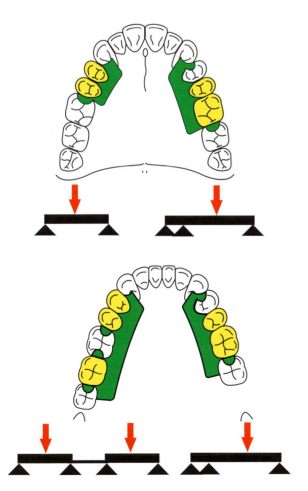

There are no problems with load distribution

Support

The aim is to rely entirely upon tooth support, by means of occlusal, cingulum, or possibly incisal rests.

Problems encountered:

- the need to prepare the teeth, to accept rests without creating occlusal interferences
- in the case of abutment teeth which have lost periodontal support, it may be necessary to find an alternative, adjacent tooth
- a long saddle which might overload the supporting teeth—reduce the loading by using a narrow occlusal table for the saddle

Connector selection

If the oral hygiene and dental condition are adequate, a cast metal connector is to be preferred (high strength, minimum bulk and least tissue coverage). In this case selection can be made from the range of options as shown on the next two pages:

(A) Upper denture

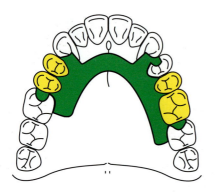

Anterior bar

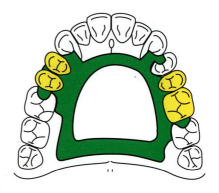

Ring

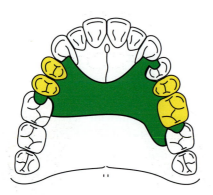

Middle bar

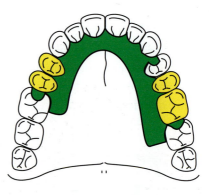

Anterior plate

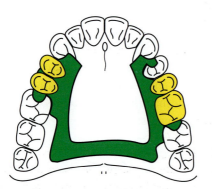

Posterior bar

(B) Lower denture

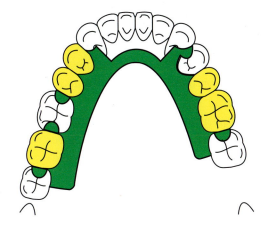

Lingual (or sublingual) bar

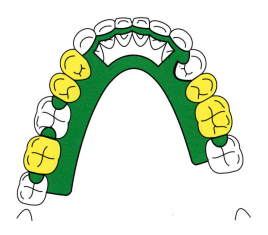

Lingual bar with accessory connector

(C) Dental bar and plate connectors

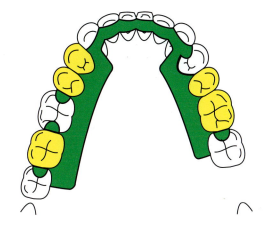

Dental bar

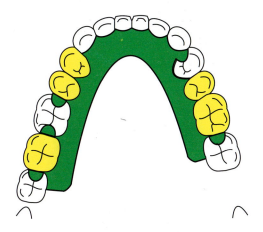

Lingual plate

Note that if only one saddle is needed, the connector will be required to cross the mouth to achieve retention, since unilateral dentures, unless locked into position (Chapter 3.10), are generally regarded to be a swallowing or inhalation hazard.

If the oral hygiene and oral state are very poor, with the early prospect of further tooth loss, there may be a case for selection of an acrylic connector (palatal or lingual plate), despite the lesser strength, greater bulk, and tissue coverage. This possibility is discussed in Section 3.

Retention

Generally, for bounded saddle designs, retention will depend principally on clasps. The casts, already surveyed, will reveal suitable locations for occlusally or gingivally approaching clasps. Clasp distribution has been discussed earlier (Chapters 1.7 and 1.8). For this class of denture it is usually possible to achieve sufficient direct retention, unless:

- patients object to the aesthetics
- the occlusion does not permit
- there are previously crowned or otherwise restored teeth which inhibit clasp placement

Here are two examples of directly retained dentures. The red lines pass through the tips of the clasps, showing that in both cases the denture base is well held in place.

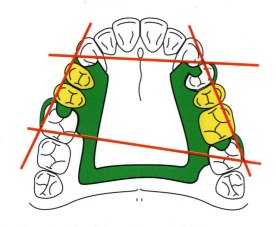

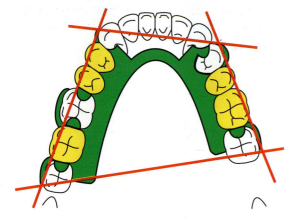

Directly retained as the bulk of the dentures lie within the area held by the clasps

Indirect retention may be needed if there are restraints on clasp placement, so that it is not possible to include all of the denture base within the 'box' formed by the red lines.

Review of the provisional design

The important aspects are:

- does the design avoid the creation of occlusal interferences? If not, can the problem be solved either by tooth preparation or by alternative component location?
- are support and retention adequate, without being excessive (for example, are there more components than really needed, leading to greater oral hygiene problems)?
- is the design as hygienic as possible, especially with regard to gingival margin coverage and encroachment?
- does the design compare well with, or improve on, a previous denture?

When satisfied on all these counts (and after discussion with the patient), a definitive design can be drawn on paper, and on the study cast. Any tooth preparation needed should be carefully identified for completion before recording the final impression(s) using special trays.

Conclusions

This chapter should have enabled you to develop a draft design for the Kennedy III case (bounded saddles only). Provided that abutment teeth are sound, this is often the most satisfactory type of design, as the denture base is usually supported by the teeth alone. Therefore the foundation upon which the denture rests is uniform.

> **Some points to remember**
>
> Once you have developed a draft design, it is essential to review the implications of the design. This was considered more fully in Chapter 1.10, but some points to consider are:
>
> - check against the articulated study casts, to look for possible occlusal interferences
> - assess carefully the oral hygiene implications
> - can the design be simplified without detracting from the prospects of success?
> - how does your design compare with the patient's past experience of partial dentures (if any)

Designing for Kennedy class I and II dentures (bi/unilateral free-end saddles)

Kennedy class I and II designs require consideration of the problems of free-end saddles. The particular difficulties are:

- provision of support during functional loading of the saddle (denture rocks)
- creation of adequate retention

Both of these are a direct consequence of the absence of posterior abutment teeth.

Saddle design

The anterior/posterior support disparity leads to a risk of damage to either the anterior abutment, or the muco-periosteum (or mucous membrane) under the free-end saddle. It is essential to minimize the functional loading, especially if the saddle is opposed by the natural teeth of the other jaw.

Methods available are:

- the use of narrow posterior teeth
- omit one or even two posterior molars (unless needed to occlude with opposing natural teeth)
- occasionally, it may be wise to avoid provision of a saddle, or even advise against denture provision altogether (see Section 3)
- cover soft tissue widely to reduce load concentration and extend the base onto areas that provide the greatest support, for example the buccal shelf for a mandibular denture

Support

The anterior end of a free-end saddle must be tooth supported, otherwise functional load will displace (compress) the saddle tissues adjacent to the abutment tooth and damage its gingival tissues ('gum stripping').

An occlusal or cingulum rest is therefore required. It is generally agreed that if the abutment tooth is a premolar or molar tooth, such a rest should be placed mesially to reduce the tilting force.

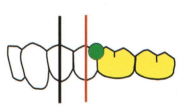

Unloaded

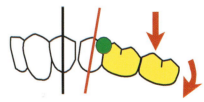

Distal rest

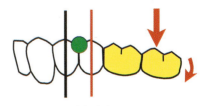

Mesial rest

To minimize the destructive forces on the abutment tooth from functional loading of the saddle, a combined rest and clasp system can be adopted (RPI system). This will be described shortly. See also Chapter 3.7 for additional techniques in relation to differential loading between teeth and tissues.

Connector selection

From the foregoing it can be seen that support will usually be provided by a combination of tooth (anteriorly) and tissue (posteriorly). This will influence connector selection.

For the upper denture optimum tissue support can be provided by palatal coverage; this constitutes a significant case for the use of a plate connector.

For the lower denture there is no such option, the best tissue support is that of full extension into the functional sulcus depth (posteriorly) and on to the retromolar pad and the buccal shelf of the mandible.

For both upper and lower dentures, there may need to be further consideration of connector selection when retention is considered (where clasps are to be placed).

Retention

Just as there is a problem of support of a free-end saddle, so there is a need for concern with retention. Clasps can be placed on abutment teeth, which will retain the anterior region of the saddle, albeit at the cost of further stressing of the abutments. For this reason the position of the clasp and the way in which it reaches the undercut have to be carefully thought out (Chapter 1.7). However care needs to be taken to create adequate retention of the posterior region.

Methods available:

- minimize displacing forces by carefully shaping the polished surfaces of the saddles (muscle action)
- make an upper denture as light as possible
- **use indirect retention** (Chapter 1.8). This requires detailed consideration

Indirect retention: upper denture

Clasping of an abutment tooth (Kennedy class II) or abutment teeth (Kennedy class I) does not prevent downward displacement of the distal end of the saddle(s). Contact of the denture with structures, as far anterior as possible from the clasp axis, to act as a fulcrum, makes the clasps effective in achieving posterior retention.

Possible anterior contact to provide indirect retention:

- cingulum rests, ideally on central incisors
- the anterior rest on the abutment of a contralateral bounded saddle may provide this in a Kennedy class II case
- horseshoe connector covering all cingula (but also covers gingival margins which may be periodontally disadvantageous)
- anterior palatal bar connector, but resting on soft tissue, is less effective than tooth contact
- use of palatal coverage, usually an acrylic resin plate (which can avoid gingival coverage), is effective and gains additional retention from the larger area covered. Disadvantage: bulky and relatively weak (a cast metal equivalent is heavier)

The only difference between the following two illustrations is the addition (overleaf) of a cingulum rest. This shifts the fulcrum forward, from the second premolar to the incisor, so improving the indirect retention.

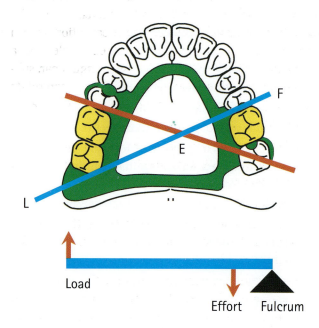

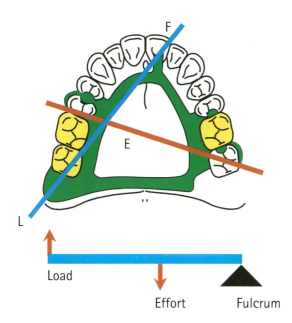

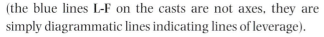

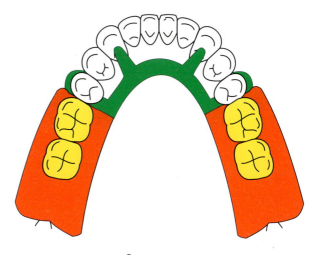

Cummer arms
(indirect retainers)
also supplying tooth support

(the blue lines **L-F** on the casts are not axes, they are simply diagrammatic lines indicating lines of leverage).

Indirect retention: lower denture

During mastication, adhesive forces (from sticky foods) will tend to rotate (displace) the free-end saddle(s) about the abutments. As in the case of the upper denture, anterior contact is needed to create indirect retention. For the lower denture, however, the only practical option is tooth contact. This strongly influences connector selection: a bar connector lying only on soft tissue (lingual bar, sublingual bar) becomes unacceptable because it can rotate deeper into the sulcus as the free-end saddle lifts.

Possible options:

- a lingual bar or a sublingual bar but add finger rests ('Cummer arms') on to the cingulum of one or both canines or central incisors
- a dental bar
- a lingual plate—cast metal is better than acrylic resin—but suffers from the disadvantage of wider gingival coverage
- use a lingual/sublingual bar but add a second connector around the cingulum area (sometimes called a continuous clasp). Disadvantage: unhygienic and may be poorly tolerated by some patients because of tongue interference

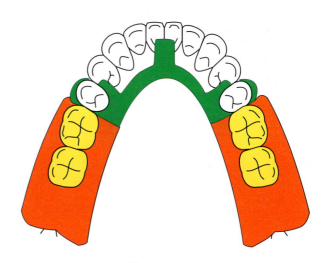

Cingulum rests
(indirect retainers)
tooth support from first premolars

A combined support and retention system for free-end saddles—the RPI system (Chapter 1.7)

To protect the abutment and its supporting structures which are vulnerable to damage, a system of rests and clasps has evolved. This is the **Rest, Plate and 'I' bar** system.

Note: The RPI elements, although cobalt chromium, are coloured blue to distinguish them from the rest of the denture base (green).

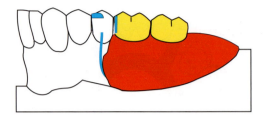

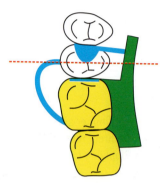

Occlusal view

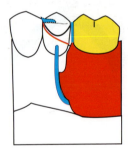

Buccal view

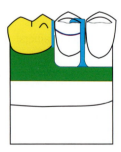

Lingual view

undercut (in most cases). The plate on the distal side of the abutment tooth is vertical, only touching the tooth surface at the vertical survey line so that any movement of the saddle towards the tissues allows the plate to move into the undercut area without applying a torque to the tooth.

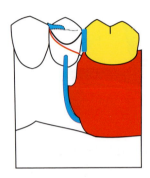

At rest

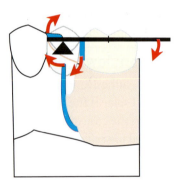

Rotation about the fulcrum

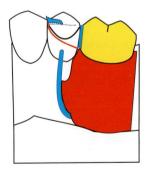

Loaded saddle

From the diagrams it can be seen that that, on loading the free-end saddle, it is accepted that the denture is going to rotate about the distal edge of the mesial occlusal rest. The gingivally approaching 'I' bar is placed on that axis and therefore the active tip will show minimum movement, and what movement it does make will be further into the

Review of the provisional design

The process of trying to reach an acceptable outcome with a difficult situation will have identified the need for careful design. The eventual design will contain compromises such as requiring significant loading of abutment teeth to create acceptable support and retention.

However, even with great care in the design of support and retention, a free-end saddle denture is fundamentally mechanically unstable. Load applied anteriorly, on the tooth supported end of a saddle, will depress the abutment tooth by a small amount (of the order of 0.1 mm). In contrast, loading posteriorly at the tissue supported end will displace (compress) the underlying mucosa by much more (around 1–2 mm, variable). Techniques occasionally used to address this dilemma are mentioned in Section 3. Furthermore alveolar resorption, possibly accelerated by loading, will progressively increase the tendency for posterior sinking. An important aspect of free-end saddle dentures is the arrangement of periodic assessment during use.

Remember that any bounded saddles present give 'modifications' (see Chapter 1.3)

Conclusions

Free-end saddles, whether bilateral (Kennedy class I) or unilateral (Kennedy class II) pose problems of support and retention. These can be minimized by appropriate saddle design and carefully located components for indirect retention and support (Chapters 1.8 and 1.9).

Some points to remember

Free-end saddles usually:

- limit selection of connector design, especially for the lower denture, and may entail greater gingival margin coverage than is desirable
- abutment teeth may be threatened by either gum-stripping or by overload
- a patient provided with free-end saddle denture(s) should attend for regular review
- you may wish to consult Chapter 3.7 for some more advanced solutions which have been devised to help with free-end saddle denture design
- do your best to refine your design

2.6 Designing for Kennedy class IV dentures

Anterior tooth loss creates the greatest incentive for a patient to seek replacement

As originally defined, this classification of missing teeth constitutes the need for a single anterior saddle, technically crossing the mid-line. The classification includes, however, a range of possibilities. At one extreme, missing central incisors would require a short saddle, while at the other extreme a large saddle would be needed if, for instance, only molars were retained (bilaterally). Patient expectation of aesthetics and stability are important factors in the design of these dentures.

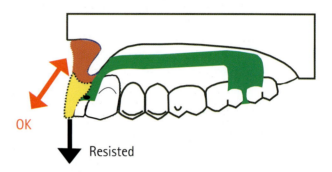

> **Remember** that *any* other saddle present will alter the basic classification to a I, II, or III (see Chapter 1.3).

Saddle design for a few missing teeth

Positioning anterior teeth, especially in the upper arch, requires attention to tooth placement for optimum restoration of the appearance.

In addition the overbite and overjet created are important for appearance and function.

The labial flange for anterior saddles

This can make a significant contribution to saddle appearance and function:

- if there is very little alveolar resorption a pleasing appearance can be obtained by omitting the labial flange (open faced/gum fitted)
- if there is more resorption, the addition of a labial flange will enable the restoration of lip support
- if a labial flange can engage an anterior soft tissue undercut it will aid retention

Fixed prostheses

Consideration should also be given to the provision of a fixed prosthesis such as:

- adhesive bridge—less destruction of the abutments
- conventional bridge with abutment preparations
- implant-supported crown or bridgework

The method of choice will depend upon many factors, including:

- state of the abutment teeth and their periodontal condition
- vulnerability to trauma such as exposure to contact sports
- prospect for maintenance by the patient and dentist
- volume and quality of bone if considering implants
- economics

In the event that a denture is advised, this may on occasions be considered as a temporary solution before embarking on a more, often fixed, permanent solution or while restorative work on other teeth is completed.

Support for a short anterior saddle

The denture teeth, for example, two central incisors, will lie between the abutment teeth. Therefore, provided the occlusion permits, cingulum rests on the abutments will provide adequate support. If opposing tooth contacts leave insufficient space, tooth preparation to overcome this difficulty is preferable to allowing the saddle to be tissue supported, since this will lead to 'gum stripping' damage to the abutments, exacerbated as alveolar bone loss advances. In the following diagrams supporting rest are marked in black, so that you can identify them clearly.

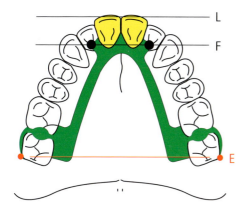

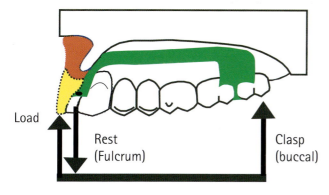

The posterior additions help stabilize the saddle, supply indirect support for the incisors, and avoid a hazard to health (inhalation or swallowing). Note the following paragraphs on connectors.

Connectors for short saddles

A short anterior saddle, on its own, would be at risk of being swallowed, or worse, inhaled. There must therefore be connectors to a more posterior region, usually molars, bilaterally (also providing indirect support and indirect retention).

Upper denture connectors

The options are:

- two cast bar connectors, (cobalt chromium is strong, hygienic and gives minimal gingival margin coverage, see above)

- horseshoe connector (metal or acrylic, less hygienic because of gingival margin coverage; acrylic resin is weak)

- palatal plate (metal or acrylic resin, metal is heavy) is only hygienic if gingival margin coverage is minimal but can be as little as that of an anterior bar connector design

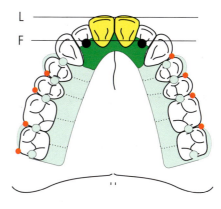

This diagram shows five possibilities from which to select connectors to carry rest/clasp elements. As the connectors are increased in length posteriorly, each increment (shown by the dotted lines indicating progressive lengthening of the denture base) increases the indirect support as the point of action of the clasps moves further away from the fulcrum. The red dots show the points of action of the clasps, on the left distally-approaching and on the right mesially-approaching clasps.

The rests supporting the **saddle** (fulcrum axis) are marked in black.

Lower denture connectors

There are fewer possibilities than for anterior upper teeth for connection of the saddle to more posterior parts of the denture:

- lingual bars or sublingual bars providing posterior connection for the saddle (cast metal, strong and hygienic)
- lingual plates (metal or acrylic resin, less hygienic, weak if made of acrylic resin)

Retention of short saddles for Kennedy IV cases

For other classifications, it has been possible to consider clasps on or near the abutment teeth. This is unlikely to be acceptable for short anterior saddles, because they would be immediately visible, especially in the upper jaw. Clasps placed more posteriorly, possibly on premolars, will be less effective. However, if there are rests more posteriorly they, together with premolar clasps, will provide indirect retention.

The occlusally-approaching clasps on the canines may not be aesthetically acceptable, whereas a gingivally-approaching clasp placed in the distal undercuts would be far less visible (see diagrams on the right).

- The anterior clasps provide retention for the saddle while the posterior clasps provide indirect support.
- The anterior rests provide support for the saddle while the posterior rests provide indirect retention.

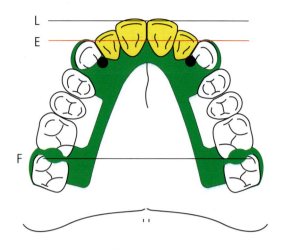

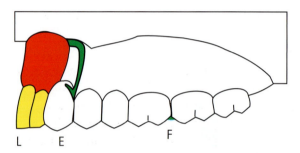

The next two diagrams should be considered as four designs, two upper (left and right) and two lower (left and right), to compare the effectiveness of the lever systems providing **indirect retention**.

Upper dentures

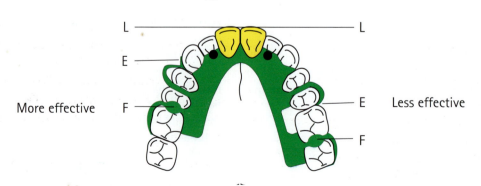

More effective   Less effective

Lower dentures

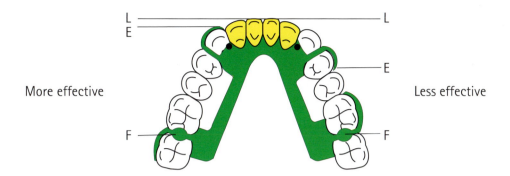

Longer anterior saddles

When more teeth are missing, problems increase.

Saddle design

The position of teeth on the saddle is important for appearance. In addition a labial flange contributes to support of the upper lip. It may be helpful to assess (but not necessarily reproduce) the original tooth positions by reference to the relatively fixed point of the incisive papilla. The labial surfaces of upper central incisors usually lie about 10 mm in front of the centre of the papilla.

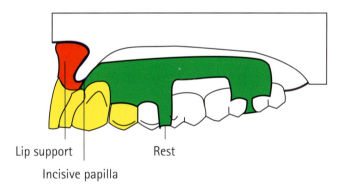

A saddle so-designed will lie on an arch which is anterior to the abutment teeth and the location of occlusal rests.

Support of longer anterior saddles

Rests are a requirement. However, because the saddle is in effect cantilevered forward from the rest sites, functional loading will lead to movement towards the tissues. Indirect support must be provided to prevent rotation of the saddle towards the tissues in function.

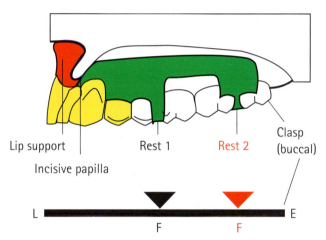

Should the lever system be insufficient to provide complete indirect support for the saddle, then the denture will rock about the rest nearest to the saddle. If rest 1 is present there is protection for the gingiva of the second premolar but there will be considerable rocking if the denture moves in function. (If rest 2 alone is present there is less protection for the gingiva of the second premolar but there will be less rocking if the denture moves in function.)

Connectors for long saddles

The longer the saddle, the shorter the connector and the less scope for avoiding gingival margin coverage. Therefore the probability increases of needing to use a horseshoe connector (preferably in metal) or palatal coverage (which could be acrylic resin) for an upper denture, or a lingual plate for the lower.

Retention of the longer saddle

Anterior clasps remain a problem, but the main aim must be to place the retainers as far forward as appearance constraints allow, together with distal extension of the connectors carrying rests (or at least contacting posterior teeth well above the survey line) to achieve the best possible indirect retention.

Here are two examples:

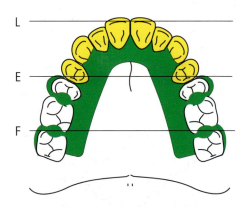

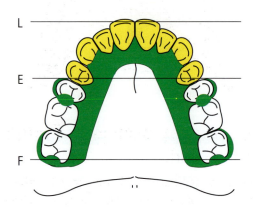

The lower diagram is more effective as the ratio of fulcrum/effort to fulcrum/displacing load is improved. Further there is a little accessory aid from the forward-facing molar clasps.

Anterior clasp placement is less of a problem for appearance in the lower jaw, although in the upper jaw it is sometimes possible to 'hide' a gingivally-approaching clasp by locating it in a distal undercut.

Review of the provisional design

Partial dentures for this situation do present problems. However, because the anterior teeth are usually better maintained, they are often retained longer than the posterior teeth.

It is necessary to employ indirect support and indirect retention in most cases; this is summarized in the next diagram:

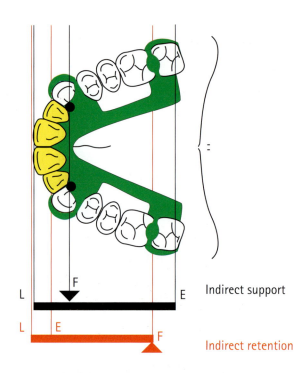

Indirect support

Indirect retention

This design shows both indirect support and indirect retention.

The lever system for each is shown so that the differing points where the fulcra and efforts are applied can be contrasted.

Aesthetically, gingivally-approaching clasps can, in general, be designed to be less obtrusive by employing distal undercuts on teeth such as canines.

As already stated, the labial flange can serve two purposes, namely restoring form and aiding retention.

There are other situations where acrylic plate dentures are employed, the upper dentures covering the palate or the lower a lingual plate. These may be the designs of choice in certain circumstances (Section 3), especially in the case of a deteriorating dentition:

- a temporary denture, while other treatment is undertaken (for example, a fixed prosthesis/periodontal therapy)
- where the saddle is so large that tissue support and tissue coverage is essential

Temporary replacement of a few teeth

An acrylic resin denture can be provided quickly and economically, but still warrants thoughtful design. The simplest (and least functional) is the 'spoon' denture.

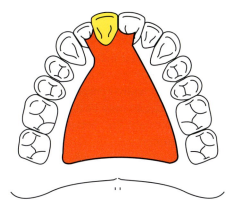

Rests essential

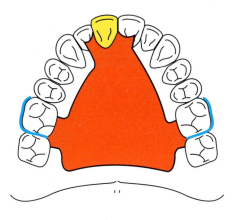

Improved retention and stabilization

The upper small saddle is tooth supported (without the cingulum rests it would be a 'gum stripper'). It is retained by tissue coverage, although a labial flange might provide some mechanical retention.

Lower down, molar contacts improve the location, and provided that the lower teeth permit, clasps provide direct retention of the denture base. Distal extension of the denture base will form a fulcrum which, acting with the clasps, will provide some indirect retention for the saddle. Note that despite the extensive palatal coverage, gingival margin coverage is no greater than it would be with a metal design, and is greatly preferable to either of the following:

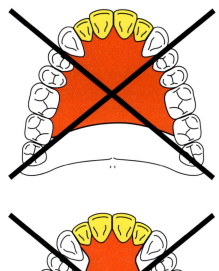

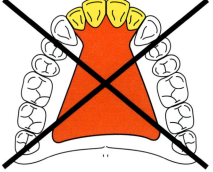

Temporary replacement of large anterior saddle

When a large saddle is needed, there may be little alternative to the use of an acrylic plate connector. This would certainly be the choice (palatal or lingual) as an interim solution to provide support and retention.

The 'temporary' nature may cover:

- restoration of remaining teeth
- consideration of implant placement to support and retain the long saddle
- incorporation of attachments into the crowns of remaining teeth
- a training period prior to progress to complete dentures

These possibilities will be discussed in Section 3. It may be the case when there are very few teeth left, that an acrylic denture may be the treatment of choice. Care should be taken to avoid a design that could damage the remaining teeth and soft tissues.

Conclusions

Although there are several options for anterior tooth replacement, including fixed prostheses, dentures with anterior saddles only are important for appearance. However these present problems of support and retention, especially if the saddle is extensive (more than two or three teeth).

Some points to remember

- Denture movement during speech or chewing can be very visible and distressing
- Indirect retention (Chapter 1.8) is usually essential and is best achieved by maximum distal extension to create a fulcrum
- Indirect support, again by maximum distal extension (but this time to provide clasping), may also be helpful (Chapter 1.9)
- Ideal anterior clasps, for indirect retention placed on abutment teeth, may prove aesthetically unacceptable although gingivally-approaching types may be less visible. (There can only be direct retention if the saddle is on a straight line between the clasps and rests on the abutments)
- Refine your design (Chapter 1.10)

Section 3

Some problems and solutions

In Section 2, we have presented a design strategy and sequence which draws upon the basic principles of partial dentures described in Section 1.

For this third section we will attempt to deal with the significant number of circumstances where difficulties present themselves, most notably in the state of the remaining dentition.

Some of the difficulties have already been identified, for instance the problem of support and retention of the free-end saddle. We will, therefore, at least introduce you to some more complex (and in some cases more advanced) solutions to this and other design problems.

Although it can become quite absorbing as a denture design develops, you must never lose sight of the fact that you are working to integrate a mechanical contrivance into a body. In so doing there are always risk factors to be considered, so before embarking on the final section of this book we would draw your attention to the following notes.

Possible risk factors associated with the wearing of partial dentures

Susceptibility to caries

- New lesions
- Lesions around existing restorations
- Root surface caries
- Risk to abutment teeth adjacent to the saddles
- Risk increased with poor salivary flow associated with some disease states or medication

Susceptibility to gingivitis and periodontal disease

- Inflammation of the gingival tissues
- Loss of attachment—pocketing, recession
- Increased mobility of the teeth
- Particular risk to abutment teeth adjacent to the saddles
- Risk likely to be increased in smokers
- Mechanical damage due to overloading of the supporting periodontal attachment

Susceptibility to soft tissue damage

- Denture induced stomatitis—denture wearing habits, oral and denture hygiene, adaptation of prostheses, role of Candida organisms, general health, possible allergic response to the denture-based materials
- Hyperplastic lesions—resulting from long-term wear of poorly fitting dentures
- Overloading of the supporting mucoperiosteal tissues
- Risk of fibrous replacement of alveolar bone on long mucosal-supported saddles opposed by natural teeth

Susceptibility of the masticatory apparatus

- TMJ dysfunction

Effects of partial dentures on plaque accumulation

- Stagnation areas in the dentition and/or on the prosthesis
- Increased susceptibility to plaque accumulation around the teeth in the same arch in which the denture is being worn
- Increased susceptibility to plaque accumulation around the teeth in the opposing arch where a denture may not be worn
- Particular susceptibility of abutment teeth adjacent to the saddles
- Increased plaque accumulation with night wear of prostheses

Prevention of disease progression when wearing partial dentures

- Oral hygiene
- Denture hygiene
- Dietary advice
- Fluoride toothpaste / mouthwashes
- Hygiene therapy and maintenance
- Smoking cessation advice
- Regular recalls

Designing partial dentures for the ageing dentition

3.1

Special consideration should be given to designing partial dentures for the elderly patient.

A number of features of the dentition of the elderly patient impact upon partial denture design. In particular we must consider general health, mobility, and self-care capability.

Economics, also, may be a significant factor in retirement years.

We will consider the questions arising from identification of a patient with a natural dentition in serious decline later, but it is worthwhile thinking about denture design for the sound, well-maintained older dentition. The following features may be found:

- tooth wear
- gingival recession, creating exposed dentine and cementum, and increased undercut zones
- sometimes progression of drift and overeruption, when permitted by earlier unrestored tooth loss. We will discuss these in some detail in Chapter 3.5

> **Abrasion:** loss of tooth substance or of a restoration, caused by wear not due to tooth contact
>
> **Erosion:** progressive loss of tooth substance by chemical processes that do not involve bacterial action
>
> **Attrition:** the loss by wear of tooth substance or of a restoration resulting from mastication or from contact between occluding or approximal surfaces

Tooth wear

You may find evidence of abrasion, erosion, and attrition. Abrasion and erosion may have created changes in tooth surfaces which we may need to contact or cover with a partial denture or its connectors. Abrasion, typically from tooth brushing, arises primarily in areas of exposed root surface, following gingival recession. This we will discuss shortly.

Erosion can, in extreme cases, also result in dentine exposure. Both abrasion and erosion create potential caries risk areas if plaque accumulation increases (in association with a partial denture).

Attrition also needs to be assessed carefully. Some wear can be expected (a 70-year-old has been using the incisors for over 60 years). Earlier tooth loss may have reduced the number of occluding teeth, and this may generally be considered to increase the potential for wear of the remainder. Furthermore parafunctional habits such as bruxism may be considered to be a significant risk factor for tooth wear.

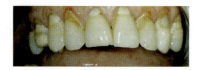

Abrasion
Note the cervical tissue loss

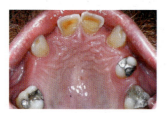

Erosion
Palatal dentine exposed

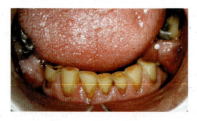

Attrition
Incisal edges worn down to dentine

Occasionally, then, you will meet a situation where there is advanced loss of crown structure, exposing coronal dentine, most visibly but not exclusively, on anterior teeth. It is tempting, but unwise and naive, to conclude that the patient must therefore be overclosed. Instead, it is quite likely that there has been compensatory overeruption, especially if the attrition rate has been relatively slow.

Clinical assessment

- There may be a good case for providing partial denture(s) to spread functional loads (and possibly reduce the rate of further attrition).
- The effect of attrition upon occlusal vertical dimension can best be assessed by measurement of the freeway space (normal range 2–4 mm).
- To increase occlusal vertical dimension beyond that available within an increased freeway space is unwise and **CERTAINLY SHOULD NOT BE CONTEMPLATED**

BY MEANS OF PARTIAL DENTURE(S) ALONE, because this would greatly increase functional loading upon supporting teeth and/or tissues. At best this would be uncomfortable, at worst damaging and there could also be undesirable effects upon muscle and joint function. There seems to be more scope to make changes to the vertical dimension by means of fixed restorations such as crowns. It would appear that the masticatory apparatus can more readily adapt to such changes than similar ones made with partial dentures alone.

- Even if some overclosure can be demonstrated, bear in mind that the patient is fully accustomed to the existing occlusal vertical dimension. The saying 'you can't teach an old dog new tricks' is a gross generalization, but contains more than a grain of valuable truth.
- There may be scope to cover the surfaces of very worn teeth with an overdenture (see Chapter 3.6).
- It might also be necessary to consider whether a fixed approach would be the most appropriate form of management, for example the use of adhesive restorations (direct/indirect composite, etc).

Gingival recession

Whether the result of a natural ageing process, or the cumulative effect of periods of gingival/periodontal inflammation, gingival recession changes the situation for partial denture design:

- as crown exposure increases, so functional root length decreases with implications for denture support in particular (see Chapter 3.6 'Improvement of the crown–root ratio')
- sulcus depth reduces, sometimes there is not enough space for a connector such as a lingual bar (a dental bar may then become more appropriate)
- undercut areas on teeth, as revealed by surveying, become deeper
- for bounded saddles, in particular, there may be deep opposing undercuts at either end of a saddle (see also Chapter 3.5 'Tilted teeth')

Gingival recession increasing the depth of opposing undercuts

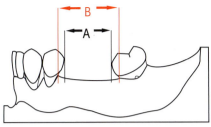

A, distance between teeth;
B, horizontal undercuts

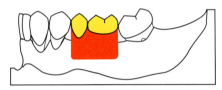

Large food trapping areas

- when gingival recession exposes cement/dentine, the presence of a denture may increase the risk of root caries (additional areas of stagnation)

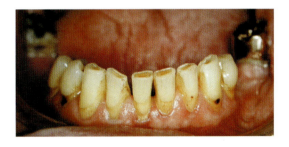

Gingival recession exposing root surfaces

- the matter of susceptibility to root caries is important, but especially so, if there is evidence of a reduced salivary flow, commonly associated with drugs prescribed for medical conditions

The design sequence applied to the healthy elderly dentition

When you embark upon the design sequence set out in Chapter 2.3, for an older patient the following should be given special consideration.

Saddle location and design

- Select sites for tooth replacement to enhance function, noting carefully the success or failure of previously provided dentures.
- Provide support as usual but beware of occlusal and cingulum rest placement to avoid interference with the occlusion (is tooth preparation necessary?). Bear in mind reduced bone support.
- Where there are deep undercuts, try to make the areas as hygienic as possible.

More marked tilting of the cast during surveying may help identify a better path of insertion (see Chapter 1.4). A so-called, self-cleansing pontic (next page) is a possible option for a posterior-bounded saddle (tooth supported), especially in the lower jaw where the saddle will be less visible.

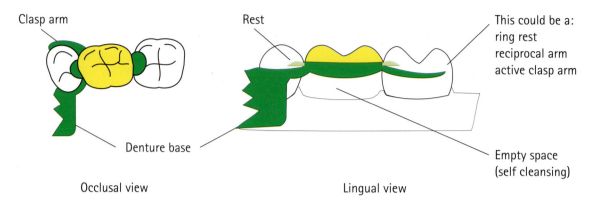

Clasp arm

Rest

This could be a:
ring rest
reciprocal arm
active clasp arm

Denture base

Empty space
(self cleansing)

Occlusal view

Lingual view

The self-cleansing pontic, well separated from the tissues, avoids stagnation and does not cover the gingival margins

Connector selection

The normal selection process but:

- assess previous experience and consider a repeat prescription if an earlier denture has proved to be non-damaging and well tolerated
- keep clear of risk areas whenever possible (for instance, does gingival recession limit sulcus depth for lingual bar connectors)
- when there are many missing teeth, and there is a need for long free-end saddles, plate designs may be the best option (palatal and lingual)

Retention

Altered undercut areas and associated exposed root tissues need to be considered:

- use more flexible materials for clasps if deeper undercuts are to be used, such as stainless steel
- avoid clasp location which may lead to plaque accumulation on the adjacent risk areas (this may contraindicate gingivally-approaching clasps, and indeed the RPI system, since both produce areas which are difficult to clean)
- indirect retention continues to be of great value (see Chapter 1.8)

Conclusions

The ageing dentition may present features that have to be considered specifically in relation to partial denture design. Features such as gingival recession and tooth wear may influence the type of components that can be placed on the prosthesis. Furthermore elderly people may encounter more difficulties in maintaining an acceptable level of oral hygiene and this should be considered when planning the type of partial denture required.

Some points to remember

Special care should be taken when there are worn teeth, exposed cementum and dentine, difficulties with self care and possibly reduced tolerance of new features. Some specific points are as follows:

- do not increase the occlusal vertical dimension indiscriminately
- avoid creating additional stagnation areas when designing partial dentures
- if an earlier denture has been successfully worn and not resulted in damage to the oral tissues, consider using a similar prescription again

New partial dentures for residual dentition in poor condition 3.2

Strategies for management of a patient with a neglected dentition.

You will be confronted, from time to time, by the patient whose remaining natural dentition is in poor condition, often as a consequence of neglect of self care and professional help. Existing partial dentures may have contributed to the deterioration.

The first step is to instigate such remedial care as the patient will accept. On occasions, you will be surprised by the patient's response, for instance the prospect of being rendered edentulous may lead to a remarkable transformation in the patient's attitude towards dental care. Oral hygiene instruction, periodontal treatment and tooth restoration may rectify the situation, and you may then be able to follow in full the principles presented in the chapters of Section 2.

For other patients, it may be necessary to anticipate further tooth loss, and plan accordingly. It is accepted for these patients that such dentures would be of a transitional nature and may well need to be modified as circumstances change.

The denture design should be appropriate to the circumstances.

- Choose relatively simple designs, possibly using acrylic resin connectors to facilitate addition of teeth as extractions are needed.
- As far as possible provide support and retention from several sources, probably including soft tissues.
- Certainly, try to avoid heavy reliance upon particular teeth for support and retention, from rests and clasps,

in case the teeth in question soon become unsaveable, when loss of these components will detract from proper function of the denture. In any case, select the soundest teeth to provide support and retention.

- Try to retain sufficient opposing natural tooth contacts to give a precise intercuspal position.

Conclusions

It is vital to emphasize to the patient what you expect to happen, so that there can be no illusions as to the longevity of the remaining dentition and the new denture(s). This will prepare the patient for future tooth loss and the additions when needed (Chapter 3.3). Clearly, too, you should stress the importance of regular review of the situation.

Some points to remember

Maintenance of a residual dentition is sometimes impossible. Partial dentures, using a simple design, may provide a useful *training* experience, assisting in the *transition* from the dentate to the edentulous state. Some specific points are as follows:

- denture designs should be kept as simple as possible
- the need for further treatment should be made very explicit to the patient

3.3 Additions to existing partial dentures

Patients with partial dentures occasionally need to lose more teeth. How can this be managed?

If, as happens, one or more of the natural teeth fails, it may be necessary to arrange for extraction. At least as a temporary measure, it is often possible to add replacement(s) to an existing denture, especially if the latter is both in good condition and is of a design which facilitates addition.

There are three potential problems:

- in the majority of cases, it is necessary for the patient to surrender the denture for laboratory work to attach new teeth
- the tooth requiring extraction may carry components critical to the satisfactory function of the denture (for instance, an occlusal rest, clasp, or indirect retainer)
- some denture designs may present mechanical difficulties in attaching additional teeth

Timing of extractions and additions

These are two ways in which the process can be organized.

- Extract the tooth, allow some healing (usually about 3 months), then arrange the clinical and laboratory procedures to make the necessary addition. This is likely to be the preferred technique where loss of the tooth would not have an effect on the appearance.
- Prepare the denture, with the added tooth prior to the extraction. This would be termed an 'immediate' or 'immediate replacement' addition.

In both the above plans, the patient must undergo impressions and occlusal recording, and then surrender the denture to the laboratory. This may be unacceptable to the patient, especially if the denture already carries replacement anterior teeth. In this event there is little alternative to the provision of a new immediate replacement denture (Chapter 3.4).

In any event, addition of teeth soon after extraction is likely to be of a temporary nature, since healing and alveolar bone remodelling will necessitate further work. A redesigned denture may even be necessary to utilize appropriate support, retention, and oral hygiene.

Loss of essential components carried by the extracted tooth

It may be necessary to arrange different plans to maintain support and retention, especially if the tooth to be lost is an abutment tooth carrying a rest and/or clasp. Of these, provision of retention is probably the most important, as without it the denture may be unusable. A simple remedy is to add a stainless steel clasp to the tooth which has now become the abutment. The new clasp can readily be included in the new acrylic saddle or saddle extension.

A particular difficulty arises when a tooth supported and retained denture (Kennedy III) has to become a Kennedy II by the loss of a distal abutment. Here, the saddle extension should be modified to follow the free-end saddle guidelines (Chapter 2.5) at the same time as the tooth addition is carried out.

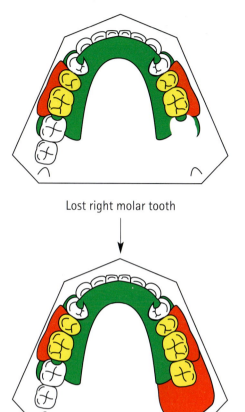

Lost right molar tooth

Addition making the free-end saddle

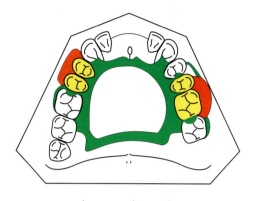

Lost anterior teeth

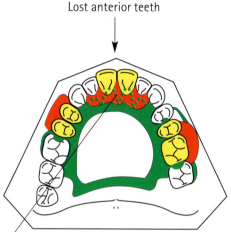

Loops of cobalt chrome wire
added to denture base

Retention aided by soldered wires

Attachment of additional teeth to the denture

There can be mechanical difficulties in attaching additional teeth to some, but not all, partial dentures:

- loss of an abutment tooth can be remedied simply by attaching the new artificial tooth to the adjacent original saddle
- loss of a tooth not adjacent to an existing saddle can be a mechanical and design problem. If the nearest connector is metal (cobalt chromium) it will be necessary to create an attachment for the new tooth, probably in acrylic resin, which will be bulky, less hygienic and possibly weak.

> **Reminders**
> - decide whether the addition can be satisfactorily achieved
> - discuss 'immediate' or later addition
> - arrange continuity of retention, and support as far as possible

Overdentures

Extraction of further teeth, for a patient who has already lost a number of teeth, should not be undertaken lightly. An alternative, involving retention of the root of the tooth, and provision of an *overdenture* (supported, and possibly retained, by the root surface) will be described and discussed briefly in Chapter 3.6. This procedure is most appropriate when the root is healthy but the crown defective.

Conclusions

Certain types of partial denture can be modified easily if it is necessary to remove any of the remaining natural teeth. Additions are most straightforward where the new denture tooth and flange can be attached to adjacent acrylic resin. The addition of a denture tooth to an existing cobalt chromium based denture can be technically challenging if the position is not adjacent to an existing saddle. This may mean that it would be more appropriate to make a new denture rather than make an unpredictable modification to the original prosthesis.

Some points to remember

There are advantages to arranging additions of further teeth to an existing denture, especially if the latter is in good condition and well tolerated. There are potential problems mainly with the mechanical attachment of the new teeth, and with loss of important components, such as clasps which acted upon the tooth to be extracted. Some specific points are as follows:

- additions can be made either by the natural teeth being extracted or because they are modified into overdenture abutments
- where a denture has been modified because of the need to extract a natural tooth, alveolar remodelling may mean that further amendments are required at a later stage

Residual dentition with poor prognosis

There are sometimes situations where there is no alternative treatment to the removal of the teeth.

This is the point of no return, where the remaining teeth and/or their supporting structures are in such poor condition that extraction is the only course of treatment.

This condition is most likely to have come about by:

- neglect
- failed remedial treatment
- disease
- change of diet
- conditions due to systemic imbalance, such as diabetes

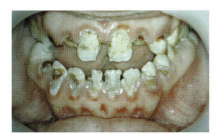

Catastrophic dental caries

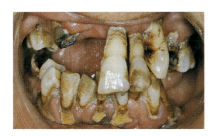

Periodontal disease

In such circumstances the decision to remove the remaining teeth will be that of the patient and the dentist.

The patient may wish to be rid of the teeth or wish them to be retained having suddenly realized their value.

You will have to use your clinical judgement to advise on the state of the dentition, taking into consideration the attitude of the patient.

The patient may or may not already have a partial denture(s).

In any event the treatment plan is to render the patient edentulous and provide complete dentures.

We can achieve this in the following ways, depending on the number and distribution of the remaining teeth:

- fit partial denture(s), to be converted later to complete dentures
- remove the worst teeth, fit a partial denture to be converted later to a complete denture
- remove the posterior teeth, fit a partial denture to be converted later to a complete denture
- provide immediate complete replacement dentures for all the remaining teeth

Much will depend on the patient's circumstances. For instance a person working on an oil rig, and so out of the public eye for extended periods, may be quite happy to be rendered edentulous and wait 3 months or so, for healing to take place, before being provided with complete dentures. On the other hand a clergyman must be confident in the pulpit that the dentures are under control and would therefore need a partial denture, on which to learn muscular control, for later conversion to a complete denture.

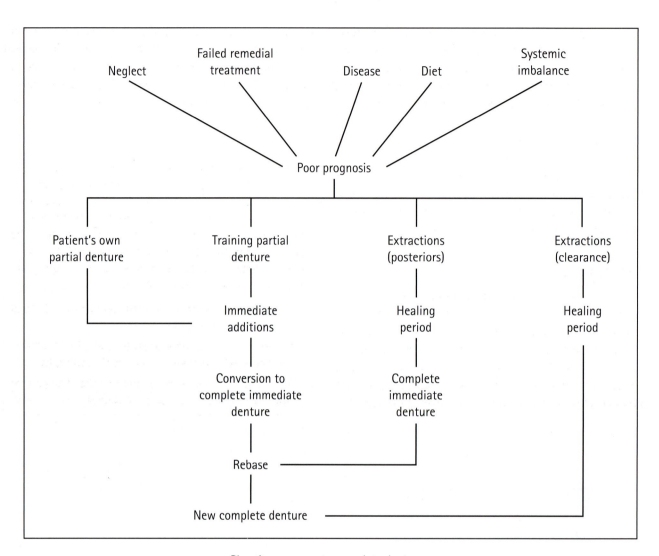

Planning progress to complete dentures

This can be shown diagrammatically as above.

Partial dentures in all these cases are of the simplest design. There need be no concerns as to gingival damage as the denture is temporary and in all probability will have more teeth added due to further tooth loss.

The type of case we will follow and recommend is that where a partial denture(s) is provided as a training appliance for complete dentures.

The decision has been made that the remaining teeth are to be removed and the patient be provided with complete dentures. In the meantime partial dentures will be fitted so that the patient can become accustomed to wearing and controlling dentures. Such dentures are constructed in acrylic and additions can be easily made if there is further tooth loss.

A simple acrylic partial denture (immediate for some teeth if necessary) is constructed, with fully extended lingual, labial, and buccal flanges rather than using 'gum fitted' (open face) anterior saddles*. There is no need for rests or clasps and in the lower denture, a lingual plate connector covers most of the lingual surfaces of the lower

* On conversion to a complete denture, a gum-fitted appliance does not retain well as the border seal is incomplete. Further, as alveolar resorption progresses, what contact there was between the gum-fitted anterior teeth and the ridge may become lost.

incisors (if present)[†]. However it may be helpful, if it is the patient's first experience of a partial denture, to use simple stainless steel clasps as a temporary aid to retention.

Once the patient is comfortable with the use and control of the denture, it can be converted into a complete denture.

Of course, it is possible to make a new complete immediate insertion denture after a training denture but conversion of the training denture is the better choice as the patient has already adapted to the exact shape of the denture and flanges. A new denture would not be the same as far as the neuromusculature is concerned.

Conclusions

The transition from a partially dentate to an edentulous state is, for many patients, a major change. The way in which this is managed will depend on the state of the remaining teeth and whether any are causing discomfort. Although some kind of transitional denture may be the preferred option for treatment, this may not always be possible. On occasions it may be necessary to extract the remaining teeth as quickly as possible and construct complete dentures after sufficient time for healing. The patient would of course then be without any natural teeth or dentures for a period of time and would have to clearly understand why it was necessary to proceed in this way.

Some points to remember

When there is no other treatment apart from the removal of the remaining teeth, there must be a planned progression to the provision of complete dentures. The extractions are most likely to be in two stages to preserve aesthetics, with a healing period to allow the posterior alveolar ridges to accept the loading of temporary partial/complete dentures (usually 3 months). Some specific points are as follows:

- these dentures are usually constructed in acrylic resin so that they can be modified easily
- the sequence of extractions and the way in which any prosthesis will be modified need careful thought
- good communication is required so that the patient understands the sequence of treatment

---

[†] Covering most of the lingual surfaces of the lower anterior teeth gives strength to the denture and at the same time allows there to be no change in that area, as far as the tongue is concerned, when the lower teeth are extracted and replaced by artificial teeth.

3.5 Partial dentures around difficult dentitions and oral structures

In some circumstances there are localized areas of the mouth which might create some problems in the construction of partial dentures. These may be related to the position of the teeth or due to other anatomical structures. Some of the problems and solutions will be considered, such as:

- overerupted teeth
- tilted teeth
- drifted teeth
- incisal overbite and overjet
- maxillary or mandibular tori
- lesions of the soft tissues

In some circumstances the position of the teeth in the remaining dentition may present challenges in designing partial dentures. This can occur either because teeth may move to a position where there is insufficient space for a prosthesis or because of the particular way that the maxilla and mandible are related. This chapter will explore some of these issues and suggest thoughts as to how partial denture design can take account of this.

Overerupted teeth

Teeth which are unopposed can in certain circumstances move because the physiological mechanisms of eruption become reactivated. We have already alluded to this previously in the discussion related to tooth wear. Teeth which overerupt can create significant problems for denture design. In many patients who are partially dentate, there is little evidence to suggest that unopposed teeth will overerupt. However in others, it seems clear that unopposed teeth have moved over time. There is still no clear way of predicting which teeth will have a greater potential to overerupt. Clearly there are biological factors operating of which we have very little understanding.

Problems created by overerupted teeth

- Disruption to the occlusal plane. The occlusal plane may be irregular in height and there may be steps between the denture or natural teeth with the over-erupted teeth. Where severe this may make mastication less efficient.

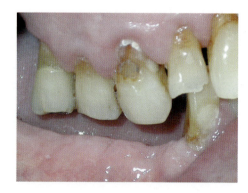

Overerupted teeth resulting in disruption of the occlusal plane

- Not enough space in the saddle area opposing the overerupted tooth to get a sufficient thickness of the denture base material. This would result in the denture being liable to fracture.

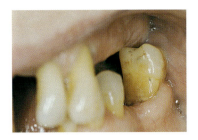

Limited space for maxillary denture

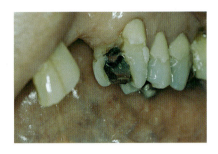

Wear facet on a premolar tooth

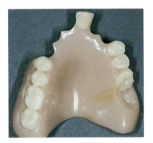

Fractured acrylic in the posterior region

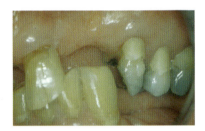

Occlusal interference from an opposing tooth

- In some circumstances the tooth may be directly in contact with the opposing ridge and there is no space at all in which a prosthesis can be placed. If such a prosthesis is constructed at an increased vertical dimension, it will often result in considerable trauma to the supporting tissues as it is heavily loaded during function. It is always dangerous to encroach on the free-way space, and to exceed it, as you should know, can be disastrous.

- They may result in occlusal interferences with the opposing dentition. The patient may change their chewing pattern which can sometimes lead to problems elsewhere in the arch, for example, tooth wear in a more anterior region or joint/muscular problems

Design solutions for overerupted teeth

In some circumstances it may be possible to work around overerupted teeth and accept that an uneven occlusal plane may result. It would appear that patients can function around uneven dentitions, but it is not known how their functional activities are compromised. Providing the disruption to the occlusal plane is not severe, this may be a perfectly acceptable solution. In other situations, a specific design of the denture or an adjustment to the teeth may be necessary.

- Striking plate: this is a modification to the design of a partial denture where the space for a prosthesis which is opposed by an overerupted tooth is very restricted. A denture with a cobalt chromium base can be designed so that it does not carry an artificial tooth in this area. Alternatively, where an acrylic resin-based denture is being used, a small piece of cobalt chromium material or a stainless steel cap may be embedded in the area. In both situations the very small thickness of metal required to give adequate strength may permit a partial denture to be designed around the abnormal position of the opposing tooth.

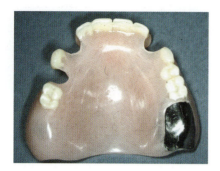

Thin striking plate to give improved strength

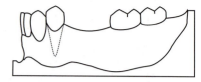

Overerupted premolar

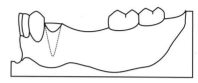

Overdenture preparation

- Reduction of the overerupted tooth: it is usually possible to make modest reductions to the opposing tooth provided it is not already crowned (in such a case there would be a danger of perforating the crown which could lead to rapid recurrent caries or fracture of porcelain). The simplest modification is the reduction of a prominent cusp, the reduction of which will create the space required for the prosthesis. However where a tooth is significantly overerupted, simple reduction of the enamel will not generate enough space. One possible solution is to reduce enough enamel and dentine from the tooth to allow it to be crowned at a much lower level. However this may involve a significant reduction of enamel and dentine, not only to bring the tooth to the correct level, but also to generate enough space for the crown itself. It would be important to consider the possible effects on pulpal health when considering reduction of this magnitude.

- Reduction of the overerupted tooth to an overdenture abutment: this may be a useful modification to the tooth as it will almost certainly create the space required for the prosthesis. It would be likely to involve elective endodontics as the pulp of the tooth would be affected by this. Furthermore, one would have to consider the implications of reducing the clinical crown on the arch of which it is a part. For example the reduction of an overerupted lower premolar tooth may create an unfavourable appearance. However this would not be a problem if the patient was already needing to wear a denture. The reduction of teeth for overdenture abutments is considered further in the next chapter.

- Orthodontic intrusion: in some circumstances it may be possible to intrude a tooth to create the space. This might be accomplished by the use of a specifically designed appliance or bite plane. However it is likely that the conditions in which such a tooth movement could be made would not arise very often, particularly when a patient may have lost a number of other teeth. Therefore for many patients this would not be a realistic treatment option.

- Extraction of the tooth: where overeruption is severe, this may be the only realistic way of dealing with the problem that has been created. In a similar way to the discussion on overdenture abutments, it would be necessary to consider the effects on the opposing arch of such tooth removal

Tilted teeth

Teeth adjacent to an edentulous space may in some circumstances tilt forward, although some lower premolars will tilt backward. This can cause difficulties in designing a partial denture. Some of the problems created are similar to those encountered with overerupted teeth e.g. irregular occlusal plane etc. However there are some additional specific issues that should be considered.

- Creation of a large undercut region adjacent to the saddle: this can create a significant problem for a bounded-saddle prosthesis where there might be a similar undercut on the abutment tooth at the opposite end. This can result in large stagnation areas around abutments where the structure of the tooth and periodontal integrity is of great importance (see also Chapter 3.1)

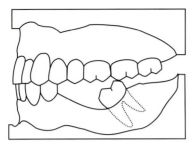

Tilted molar

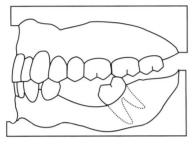

Tilted premolar and molar

- Difficulty in providing support to the prosthesis down the long axis of the tooth: an occlusal rest from a denture placed on the occlusal surface of the tooth closest to the saddle may mean that the tooth is loaded unfavourably. This can be exacerbated if there is already some periodontal attachment loss.

Short rest

- Some of the solutions for working around tilted teeth are as follows: if the position of the tooth is accepted, the patient will need to be advised of the need for excellent oral hygiene, as the junction between the prosthesis and the titled side of the abutment will almost certainly create a stagnation area which will result in significant plaque accumulation. As the tooth is tilted, in many cases there is no space conflict with an opposing dentition. For this reason it may be possible to design the occlusal rest so that a broad area of the tooth is covered. This would help in creating a more favourable loading over the whole circumference of the periodontal ligament.

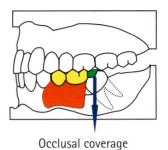

Occlusal coverage

Ring rest

- It may be possible to reduce any stagnation areas by paying close attention to the path of insertion of the prosthesis. In some circumstances it may be possible to make small modifications to the teeth to assist this. However this will have little effect on a tooth which is severely tilted.
- Orthodontic realignment of the tooth may be possible but it is unlikely that there would be many situations in a partially dentate patient where the conditions are suitable for this.
- Extraction of the tooth may need to be considered. However the effects of this on the arch as a whole need to be thought out. If the loss of the tilted tooth converted a bounded-saddle to a free end-saddle situation, this would be unfavourable. However if there was still an abutment tooth more posteriorly, then the effects would not be so great.

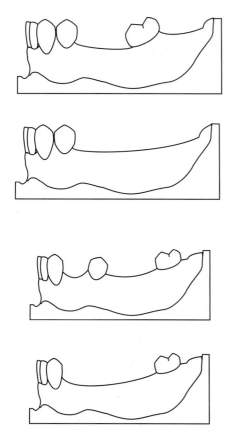

Loss of a distal abutment tooth (upper diagrams) creates a greater problem than the loss of an intermediate abutment tooth (lower diagrams)

Drifted teeth

Teeth adjacent to an edentulous space may in some circumstances drift bodily forwards or backwards into an edentulous space. The cause of this is often not clear. Teeth that have drifted away from other teeth may not necessarily cause any problems at all for partial denture design as shown below.

However some difficulties can arise when movement is in an unfavourable direction. Their resultant position may be such that there is insufficient space to locate any artificial teeth between them and other natural teeth. In such cases there are a number of possibilities.

- The prosthesis is simply designed so that it does not extend near the tooth that has drifted. The patient may have to accept a small space between the natural teeth.

- If there is insufficient space to place a denture tooth it may be possible to extend part of the denture base into it. This may be useful for example so that appropriate clasping to the adjacent teeth can be sited. It would be important that this part of the denture is designed so that stagnation areas are kept to a minimum.

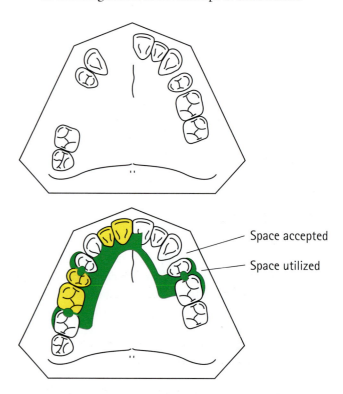

Part of a cobalt chrome connector used to fill a small space between adjacent teeth

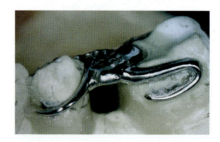

Use of a casting to restore the occlusal table where the space between the abutments is restricted (we thank Dr Mark Packer for permission to use this photograph)

- Orthodontic movement or extraction of the teeth remain possibilities as for tilted and overerupted teeth. Again, it would not be anticipated that orthodontic movement would be a commonly used treatment.

Incisal overbite and overjet

The skeletal relationships of the maxilla and mandible will to a considerable degree influence the incisal overbite and overjet. The overbite represents the vertical overlap of the upper and lower teeth, whereas the overjet represents the horizontal relationship.

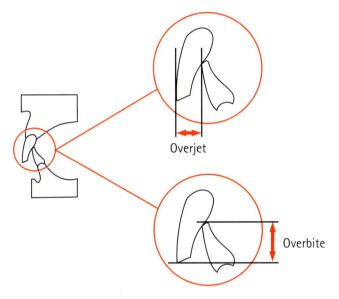

Incisal overbite and overjet, showing the relationship between the teeth

Normally the overbite and overjet will allow components of the prosthesis to be placed without interference in the creation of an acceptable appearance and harmonious occlusal relationships. Problems however can arise where there are discrepancies present.

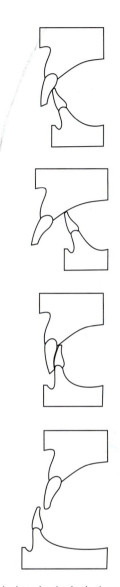

Anatomical variations in the incisal overbite and overjet

For convenience these will be considered in the following situations:

- where partial dentures do not carry artificial teeth in the anterior region
- where the replacement of anterior teeth is an important reason for providing the partial denture

Partial dentures that do not carry artificial teeth in the anterior region

Particular difficulties that can arise here are when there is an increased overbite. This can create a challenging problem when the lower incisors are in contact with the palatal soft tissues. This may cause difficulties with connector design.

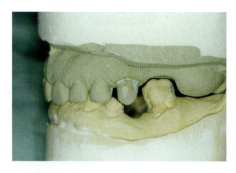

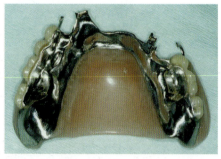

A cobalt chromium occlusal surface may be used when space is restricted

The solutions to this difficulty will depend on the pattern of tooth loss. Where only posterior teeth are being replaced, the connector can be designed so that it is clear of this area. This is the best way of managing the problem as there is no danger of the partial denture interfering with the natural occlusal relationships. This also would be a favourable design in relation to the periodontal tissues supporting the anterior teeth.

Where it is necessary to bring the connector into the anterior region (for example where there is a need to replace an anterior tooth), the properties of the denture base material in thin section will need to be considered. Acrylic resin is liable to crack or fracture when its thickness is inadequate. A cobalt chromium base plate offers superior properties in this respect. Ideally this might be the denture base material for the whole prosthesis. Alternatively, when an acrylic resin design is being used, an anterior striking plate can be embedded in the base.

Partial dentures that carry anterior artificial teeth

A deep overbite can also cause particular difficulties as follows.

- It may make the artificial teeth vulnerable to being detached or fractured from the denture base. For maximum strength the artificial teeth should be protected as far as possible by a cobalt chromium framework. Long acrylic teeth on an acrylic resin base will always be vulnerable to fracture. In certain situations it may be necessary to extend the cobalt chromium base along the palatal aspects of the artificial teeth. This protects the denture teeth from being sheared away from the base by the action of the opposing teeth. A disadvantage is that the metal backing may show through the tip of the incisors creating an unwanted greying of the appearance. In addition to this mechanical solution, some of the new adhesives offer good bonding between the materials.

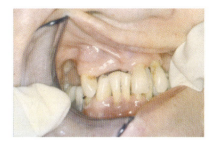

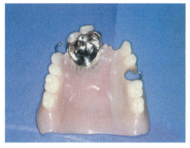

A thin cast anterior striking plate used in the case of a deep overbite (we thank Dr Pauline Maillou for permission to use these photographs)

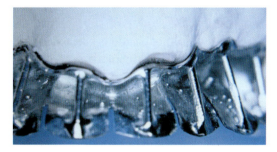

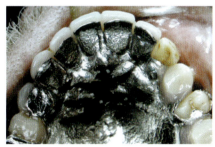

Cobalt chrome backings prevent the artificial teeth being sheared from the base

- It may result in the stability of the denture being compromised. The denture may tip during function with the posterior part of the prosthesis becoming displaced from the underlying tissues. To avoid this it is important to provide clasping as far back as possible from the saddle. This is a particular issue with the Kennedy class IV denture and has been explored in the earlier part of the book (Section 2). An alternative

approach is to attempt to reduce the overbite by appropriate positioning of the artificial teeth. This would usually result in the upper incisors being set at a higher level. However this would mean that the appearance would be compromised as the patient would show less of the teeth. Increasing the overjet raises the lip level, so sometimes a slight adjustment to both the overjet and the overbite will provide a satisfactory solution. This is a situation where the views of the patient must be sought at the try-in (trial) stage.

An increased overjet may present problems when replacing anterior teeth. The teeth will need to be positioned in a way that harmonizes an appropriate appearance, correct support for the lips and occlusal relationships that allow efficient oral function. Sometimes these objectives are mutually exclusive and compromises will have to be made.

Maxillary or mandibular tori

Tori are bony prominences that occur naturally. They are most commonly found in the mid-line of the hard palate or on the lingual aspects of the mandible. If a denture base rests on these areas, the patient may experience discomfort or pain, particularly on occlusal loading.

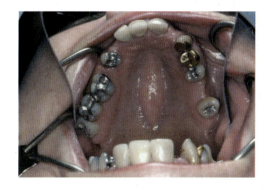

Maxillary mid-line torus

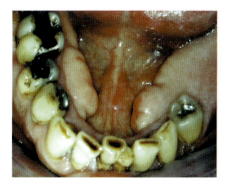

Mandibular tori in the premolar region

There are a number of possible solutions to the presence of tori, some of which involve modifications to the design of the partial denture:

- avoid covering the area with the denture base if possible. This may mean that connector design will need to be modified
- if the torus has to be covered, ensure that adequate relief is made so that the casting is not overloading the soft tissues covering the bony prominence. It is also worthwhile ensuring that the casting is made of sufficient thickness to allow further reduction if required
- rarely it might be necessary for the patient to have the tori surgically removed prior to constructing partial dentures

Lesions of soft tissues

It is not within the remit of this book to explore all of the lesions that might affect the provision of partial dentures. However in some circumstances pathological changes to the soft tissues need to be considered before embarking on denture design. Examples include denture-induced stomatitis and denture-induced hyperplasia.

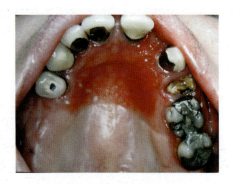

Denture-induced stomatitis

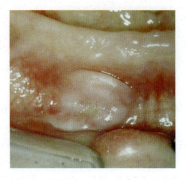

Denture-induced hyperplasia

Information from the initial examination of the patient should be assessed carefully. The usual procedure is to ensure that these conditions have been resolved before constructing new or replacement partial dentures. Occasionally it may be necessary to involve other specialists in the management of the patient (e.g. surgical removal of excessive hyperplastic tissue which would impact on the borders of the denture base). Furthermore replacement partial dentures should be designed to minimize the chances of the condition recurring.

Conclusions

There are a wide variety of situations that can occur with the natural teeth being in positions that are less than ideal for an optimum design of a partial denture. Furthermore there may be more than one aspect to this, for example, overerupted teeth may also result in occlusal interferences. When contemplating partial dentures for these patients, all the necessary information must be gathered before commencing either design or treatment. In these cases it is critical that study casts are recorded and articulated so that tooth modifications can be planned before starting the definitive treatment.

Some points to remember

Critical assessment is required for situations in which either the position of the teeth, or other structures, present challenges in the construction of partial dentures. The properties of the materials used in fabricating a denture also need to be considered in this context. Some specific points to consider are:

- can a denture be designed around a tooth with an unfavourable position or should the tooth be modified or even extracted?
- the materials that should be used where a denture has to cover an area where there is a deep overbite
- the need to resolve lesions of the soft tissues before constructing partial dentures

Overdentures and implants

3.6

An overdenture is a prosthesis that derives support from the natural teeth (or roots).
Osseointergrated implants may also be used to replace missing teeth.

An overdenture is a prosthesis that is fitted over teeth which have usually had their natural crowns reduced or removed. It has particular advantages over a conventional denture in the restoration of function and appearance. Furthermore attachments may be fitted to the roots to aid retention or support of the denture.

Occasionally overdentures are fitted over teeth with their complete clinical crowns intact. However it is more usual for these dentures to be fitted over the roots of the natural teeth where the clinical crowns have been reduced either naturally by attrition or by the dentist electively. Fitting the denture directly over the roots of teeth will often allow it to be more stable in function than if the roots were not present.

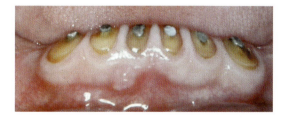

Lower anterior denture abutments

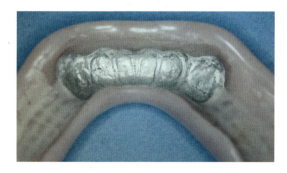

Fitting surface of the overdenture

Advantages of overdentures
Preservation of alveolar ridge form

Roots of teeth that are retained in the mouth, and have good periodontal attachment levels, will result in the alveolar bone being maintained around them. This is particularly useful where there are multiple roots that will support an overdenture, as the morphology of the ridge is likely to help with the stability of the prosthesis. It is known that the alveolar bone resorbs following loss of the teeth, and maintaining the roots will reduce this.

Furthermore it is known that roots used as overdenture abutments may prevent alveolar resorption between them. For example the retention of two canine roots in the maxilla will mean that the alveolar bone between them will be less likely to resorb.

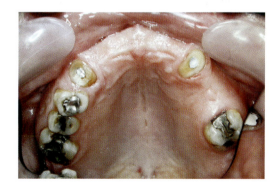

Maxillary canine roots, note the volume of alveolus

Another advantage of keeping overdenture roots is that the soft tissue profile may be maintained in a favourable way for the path of insertion of the denture. For example a maxillary canine overdenture abutment may be greatly effective in preserving a labial undercut. If the prosthesis can be designed with a path of insertion that can utilize this, then there may be considerable advantages in relation to retention and stability.

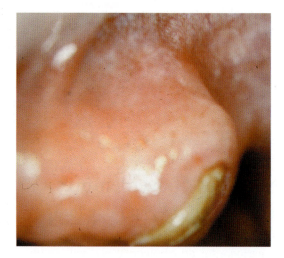

A lateral view of the maxillary canine tooth root, showing the preserved labial undercut

Optimum support for the denture

We have considered how partial dentures are supported in Section 1 of this book. In most conventional partial dentures, support is gained by means of occlusal rests. However these may not always load the tooth evenly. In contrast, an overdenture abutment can act as an ideal means of support. This is because the denture fits directly over the root and therefore permits even loading of the whole of the periodontium. Since the periodontal ligament is well adapted to take large vertical loads, there is a substantial advantage in having the overlying denture supported in this way.

The following diagrams outline how support could be made more effective by utilizing a posterior tooth as an overdenture abutment. However, due to the anatomical structure of the root face, it would nevertheless be unusual for such a tooth to be used in this way (discussed later in this chapter).

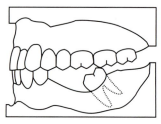

Tilted molar

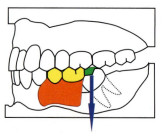

Occlusal coverage

Support for a partial denture by a large occlusal rest on the molar tooth

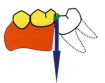

Short rest

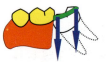

Ring rest

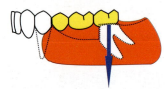

Overdenture

Greater coverage of the tooth surface may offer more idealized support

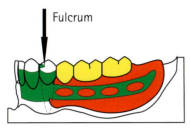

Torque applied to tooth

Rotation of the denture about the premolar on loading

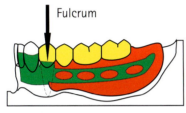

No torque on root

More favourable rotation of an overdenture

Improvement of appearance

Teeth that have become partially worn due to attrition or erosion often have a poor appearance. Taking a denture fully over the remaining part of a tooth will permit the artificial tooth to be placed so that the result is a substantial improvement in the appearance.

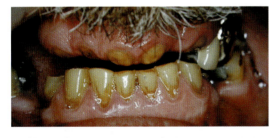

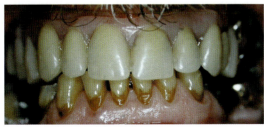

Improvement of appearance achieved with a denture overlying retained tooth roots

Improvement of the crown–root ratio

In some circumstances the clinical crowns of the remaining teeth can be very long. This often results from tooth loss in adjacent regions along with gingival recession and/or overeruption of the tooth. The clinical crown of the tooth can be quite long compared to the root of the tooth. This may also cause difficulties because the occlusal plane of the denture and the teeth may be uneven. The reduction of the clinical crown can overcome these problems, together with that of the leverage which can be applied to the root.

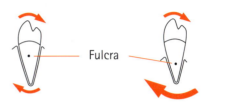

Fulcra

Torque applied to root

Preservation of sensory input from the periodontal ligament

It is known that stimulating periodontal ligament mechanoreceptors can evoke reflex changes in activity in the masticatory muscles. Furthermore these receptors, when stimulated, can evoke a reflex flow of saliva which is important during chewing. When the teeth are lost, the periodontal ligament mechanoreceptors are also lost. However if the roots of the teeth are still present, then any loading on them from the denture will continue to stimulate the mechanoreceptors that are maintained within the periodontal ligament.

Psychological benefits

By maintaining the roots of the teeth, the patient may feel that at least part of their natural dentition is being preserved. This may encourage them to stay motivated to keep the overdenture abutments.

Disadvantages of overdentures

Limitations of space

Since overdenture abutments preserve alveolar bone, their presence will mean that the denture base will not be as thick as in other edentulous areas of the mouth.

Furthermore masticatory loads will be directed through the materials of the denture base. This may result in the prosthesis being more likely to fracture. For this reason there are a number of factors to think through at the design stage. For instance, a cobalt chromium denture base may offer particular advantages in relation to strength compared with an acrylic resin-based prosthesis.

Risk of further disease of abutments

We have already explored the effects of plaque on any teeth which are in close proximity to a partial denture. Any area in which there can be stagnation and a build up of plaque can result in the initiation of further disease processes. It follows therefore that an overdenture abutment that is completely covered by a prosthesis is especially susceptible to the effects of plaque. This may manifest in two ways:

- a loss of the periodontal attachment, resulting in pocketing and ultimately an increased mobility of the tooth
- damage to the root face due to caries

A loss of periodontal attachment will mean that the tooth offers less support to the denture. Furthermore when the attachment loss becomes more severe, the tooth may need to be extracted, whereas it may be possible to repair small carious lesions to the root face. However the difficulty increases when the caries extends subgingivally. The restoration of the root face at this stage becomes far less predictable and the materials used often do not perform well in the long term.

For these reasons a decision on whether to construct an overdenture needs thought. Apart from considering the structure of the tooth itself and the periodontal support, the question of whether the patient will be able to maintain these in the long term is an important issue. The root face would appear to be particularly susceptible to caries, and so if there is a question as to whether the patient can maintain an adequate standard of oral hygiene, it may be prudent not to consider an overdenture. In particular great care should be taken if overdentures are considered in the elderly. It would be particularly important to establish whether a patient, or a member of their family or carer, can provide the necessary oral and denture hygiene required to maintain the overdenture abutments.

Factors to consider when designing partial overdentures

How much space is required over the tooth to be used as the abutment?

Although rare, there may be sufficient space between the crown of the tooth and the opposing occlusal surfaces so that the prosthesis can be designed without any reduction of the crown at all. This may occur in patients with congenital cleft palate where the growth and development of the maxilla has been compromised. In this case it may be possible to construct the prosthesis so that it fits directly over the teeth.

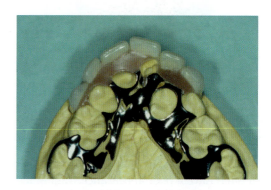

An overdenture constructed without reduction of the natural teeth

Usually it is necessary to reduce the clinical crown of the tooth. The root face is made dome-shaped just above the level and following the contour of the gingival margin.

Will tooth reduction compromise the pulpal health of the tooth?

As the amount of tooth reduction required to create an overdenture abutment is substantial, it is very likely that the pulp tissues will be damaged. For this reason it is often necessary to carry out elective endodontics to the tooth prior to reducing or removing the clinical crown.

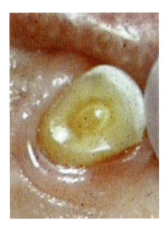

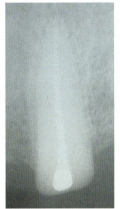

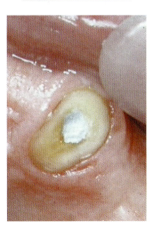

Although the pulp chamber appeared sclerosed, endodontic treatment was required

On occasion, the tooth reduction may not compromise the pulpal health. This may particularly be the case in older patients where tooth wear is already present. The pulp chamber may even be obliterated by new dentine and the root canals may become sclerosed. In such cases it may well be possible to reduce the tooth without exposing the pulp chamber.

For these reasons it is critical that a full clinical and radiographic assessment is made of any tooth that is being considered as an overdenture abutment.

Surface anatomy of the overdenture abutment

An overdenture abutment should be smooth and easy to clean. This is most easily achieved on single rooted teeth. Multi-rooted teeth present more problems. For example, the reduction of a maxillary molar with three roots can be challenging. The resulting root face could be very close to the furcation area of the tooth, or it might even be necessary to reduce the tooth even further, through the furcation area completely, and have three separate roots supporting the overdenture (on occasion, one root of a lower molar is so retained). It may be very difficult to assess before the reduction what the resulting root face would look like, and it may also be awkward to keep the subsequent abutments clean. For this reason overdentures are more usually used over anterior teeth. The root face is normally made slightly dome-shaped to blend with the gingival contours and to facilitate cleaning.

Will the overdenture abutment be susceptible to further caries or periodontal disease?

It is important to make an objective assessment about this. There are certain risk factors which may make further disease more likely. Poor oral and denture hygiene may have obvious implications. However wearing the overdenture at night may make the abutments much more susceptible to disease.

It has been suggested that coverage of the root face with a restorative material such as a metallic coping will mean that there is less surface area that could be affected by further caries. However there may still be danger at the margins of such restorations, particularly if they are located within the gingival crevice.

Is it necessary to gain additional retention from the overdenture abutment?

In some cases it is possible to place a coping carrying an attachment to which the denture can be fitted. The tooth would have to be endodontically treated in the first instance. An example of such an attachment is a disc, with a concave edge, which is fitted to a post-retained coping. A second part of the attachment is placed within the denture itself, clipping the prosthesis into place. Again, the concern about caries at the margins of the restoration is an important factor to consider. A similar system, but using magnets instead of the male and female attachments, is another method of retention that can be effective.

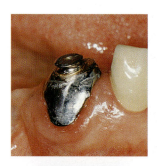

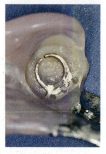

A precision attachment to retain a denture, a split ring engages a grooved counterpart on the coping

How can further disease be prevented?

Good patient selection is mandatory. In particular, it is necessary to determine that the patient is sufficiently motivated before commencing treatment. Meticulous oral and denture hygiene will be critical to future success. The use of fluoride toothpastes to clean the abutments is strongly recommended. In some circumstances it may be useful to offer further modes of fluoride application (such as fluoride gels). Finally it is necessary to recall patients at regular intervals and they should clearly understand that some maintenance will be required for long-term success.

Implants

It is not within the remit of this text to consider implants in great detail. An implant fixture is placed in alveolar bone upon which a superstructure can be constructed carrying the artificial teeth. The dental implant is sited in the bone by a surgical procedure. The process by which it becomes attached to the bone is termed osseointegration. If osseointegration is successful, the implant fixture becomes totally immobile and can be loaded without problems. It follows that an important part of the assessment of the patient is to determine whether bone is present in sufficient volume and quality in the area where the fixture needs to be sited. The patient also needs to be fit and well to undergo the surgical procedure. Factors such as a history of infective endocarditis may well contraindicate this line of treatment. Although high success rates are now reported, nevertheless this treatment method is expensive due to the cost of the components and the expertise of the clinical and laboratory staff.

In many respects implants resemble overdenture abutments and have similar advantages. They provide good support for any loading of the artificial teeth. The retentive components mean that any prosthesis should be stable during function. They even help to maintain alveolar bone. However they do not have a functioning periodontal ligament around them and there is no sensation when they are loaded. If implants are used then it is critical that the patients have very good oral and denture hygiene.

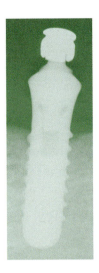
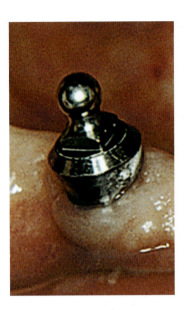

An osseointergrated implant carrying a retentive anchor to which a denture can be fitted

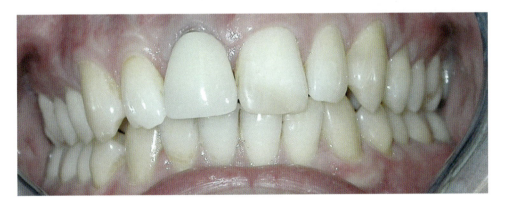

Implant-supported crown (upper right central incisor)

Implants can be used in conjunction with fixed crowns, bridges or with removable prostheses. Generally, in partially dentate patients with sufficient natural teeth remaining, it would be more likely that the superstructures are fixed to the implants and cannot be removed by the patient.

Conclusions

Overdenture abutments can provide many advantages for a patient who has to wear a partial denture. A particularly careful pretreatment assessment is required when considering this course of treatment. It is also necessary to be sure that the patient can maintain teeth/roots covered by such a prosthesis.

Implants carrying crowns or bridges may offer another solution to the restoration of partially dentate patients. As the procedure is invasive it is vital that the patient has no contraindications to surgery, so a full clinical and radiographic work-up is required. In some circumstances it may be necessary to carry out additional investigative procedures such as a CT scan to ensure that the surgeon has enough information. It is also critical that a full assessment of the remaining teeth is carried out to ensure there these are stable and have a reasonable long-term prognosis.

Some points to remember

Meticulous patient assessment is required when considering the design of an overdenture. The advantages and disadvantages of such a prosthesis should be weighed up carefully. Osseointegrated implants offer a way to replace missing teeth. In both of these treatment modalities, the patient will need to achieve a very high standard of oral hygiene. For each modality some specific points are as follows:

Overdentures

- good periodontal support is critical for any tooth being used as an overdenture abutment
- the status of the pulp needs to be considered as in some situations it will be necessary to carry out elective endodontic treatment
- as the root face may be particularly susceptible to dental caries, some thought should be given to how this can be prevented e.g. oral hygiene, fluoride, etc.
- careful assessment should be made to determine if there is sufficient space available for the denture overlying the abutment so that the denture will not be susceptible to fracture

Implants

- is the underlying bone suitable to site an implant?
- if some of the natural teeth remain, are they in a suitable condition to have a satisfactory prognosis?

Note: Roots and implants can be used for both supporting and retaining purposes.

The free-end saddle: further comments

A return to the problem of the free-end saddle, largely caused by the difference in the foundation offered by the teeth and tissues. Some attempts to minimize the damage which may be caused by movement of the denture base in function are considered.

In Chapter 2.5 we identified the particular problems of partial denture design when free-end saddle(s) are needed. Both support and retention difficulties are present. While retention of the saddle can be improved by indirect retention (quite simply, once you have grasped the principles involved; Chapter 1.8), support is more of a problem. This diagram summarizes the deficiency:

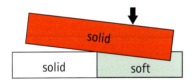

A rigid base is unstable when supported by a foundation which is not uniform

In Chapter 2.5, we described routine methods for reducing the loading of the abutment tooth and the rotational displacement anteriorly. These were:

- wide tissue coverage of the saddle base, to spread the load. This is particularly helpful with an upper denture, by extension on to the hard palate
- reduction in the occlusal table, using narrow posterior teeth and omitting one or more posterior molars

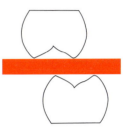

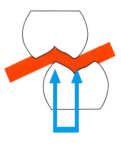

A large occlusal area has to crush a bolus

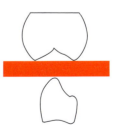

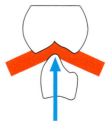

A narrow occlusal area easily penetrates a bolus

In addition to these design features, we have already emphasized the need for routine patient recall for reassessment of free-end saddle dentures. This is particularly important for lower denture wearers, because as the saddle sinks, due to progressive alveolar bone resorption, the support problem becomes exacerbated. The potential for overload and damage to abutment teeth of free-end saddles is then increased. As this occurs, it is possible to rebase the saddle area, but this has to be done very carefully to avoid detracting from the accuracy of the fit of the connector anteriorly. It may in fact be a better solution to provide a replacement denture more frequently to keep pace with alveolar remodelling, especially in the early years after tooth extraction.

Other options for management of free-end saddles

These include:

- avoid provision of free-end saddles altogether. This is particularly appropriate if adequate occlusion remains anteriorly (Chapter 3.8), and where the risk of overeruption of unopposed natural teeth can be assessed to be minimal

- design the support and retention components applied to the abutment tooth/teeth to minimize the consequences of free-end saddle movement under load, such as the RPI system, discussed in Chapter 2.5

- simulate the loaded (chewing) effect upon the free-end saddle by *displacing* ('compressing') the *tissues*, which will lie under the saddle, while making the working impression

- design a denture which allows the saddle to 'sink' into the tissues without displacement of anterior components and without rotation about the abutment, using a *flexible connector* to join the tooth supported and tissue supported units

Of these options, the first two have been detailed elsewhere. The third and fourth need further consideration.

Tissue displacement (compression)

To remind you yet again, the support problem arises because of the differential displacement ability between the natural teeth (in particular, of the abutment tooth carrying a mesial rest) and the soft tissue under the saddle. You will recall that the periodontal ligament may allow intrusion of a tooth by about 0.1 mm under load, while the areas providing tissue support may be compressed by up to 2 mm in some places.

If we could build in the extra displaceable (compressible) nature of the soft tissue when producing the denture base, the problem would be eliminated. This can be achieved, at least in theory, by using a high viscosity impression material together with pressure on the tray while making the impression. In practice this is most often attempted by means of a two-stage impression technique.

First a low viscosity overall impression is recorded. A base is constructed, which is then loaded with a high viscosity material *only* in the free-end saddle area. It is held firmly in place allowing the high viscosity material to displace and record the altered shape of the soft tissues under pressure. A material such as zinc oxide / eugenol paste would appear to have the necessary properties to enable a displasive impression of the saddle to be recorded, provided that the base fits closely to the tissues. The saddle areas of the original cast are then replaced with the new displacement version. This method is known as the Altered Cast Technique.

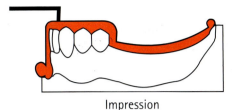

Impression

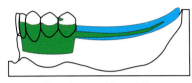

Cast base with saddle

These are sagittal sections through the crest of the lower ridge

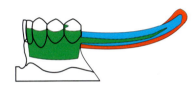

Model cut—new saddle impression

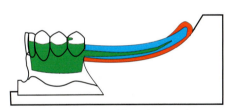

New cast poured into impression

The denture base with the new impression of the saddle area is refitted to the truncated model and cast

We hope the foregoing makes the theoretical advantages clear. However, there are some practical problems:

- the load exerted during impression-making is intended to simulate functional loads, but these are not necessarily symmetrical between left and right (Kennedy I). Also functional loads vary widely

- a denture constructed in this way presents a risk, when not loaded at rest, of producing a premature contact between the saddle and the opposing teeth as the saddles may be raised by the now unloaded tissues

- in order to keep the anterior connector and components seated, sufficient clasp retention must be provided to hold the saddle in place against the tissue recoil from the displaced state

- we suspect that enhancing tissue loading, to aid the abutment tooth, may accelerate tissue remodelling which could negate the objective of the procedure

We suspect that the altered cast technique is not used as routinely in clinical practice today as it has been in the past. Such a technique would not in any case be normally carried out for maxillary free-end saddle dentures, as the tissue support appears generally good enough to prevent instability during occlusal loading of the saddle. There is a stronger case for using it in the mandible.

Flexible connectors—the stress breaker

To remind you, yet again, the problem we seek to overcome is the disparity between tooth and tissue support:

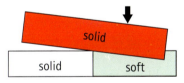

If it were possible to arrange a separation between the tooth and tissue components, the potential excess abutment tooth loading might be eliminated:

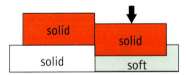

If the tooth-supported and tissue-supported parts of the denture were to be separate, there would be no instability

The ideal situation would be to share loading, avoiding over-stressing either hard or soft tissues. Look at the next mechanical drawings:

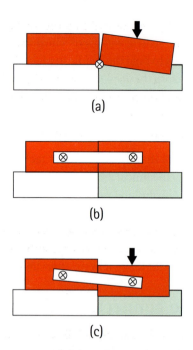

(a)

(b)

(c)

Here a simple hinge (a), or twin hinges (b, c) allow different degrees of freedom for the transmission of functional load. In (a) loads on the anterior saddle would be largely carried by the abutment; in (c) the abutment would not be loaded.

However, if instead of a hinge we used a flexible connector, we might achieve a sharing of the load:

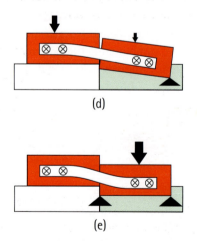

(d)

(e)

At first there is a simple bend in the connector;
further loading causes an 'S' bend as the posterior
end cannot sink further into the tissues

In (d), light loads are applied, especially distally; heavier forces generate a more complex bending of the connector and different force distribution (e).

Conversion of this mechanical theory into a practical denture design is shown diagrammatically:

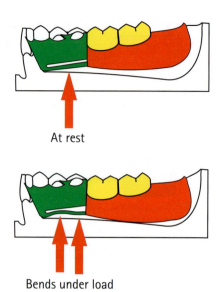

At rest

Bends under load

However, if flexible connectors, as above, were to be the only connection between the anterior section and the saddle, the connector could also bend laterally or twist allowing the saddle to move in unwanted directions, which would be intolerable. These unwanted movements would therefore have to be controlled by adding a further component:

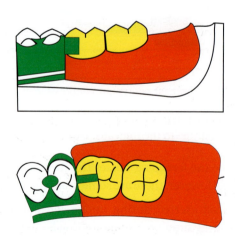

Stabilizing the free-end saddle against undesirable movement

Here a 'fin' has been made on the casting which will fit into a slot prepared in the artificial tooth. This will allow vertical movement of the saddle relative to the rest of the denture base, but will not permit lateral or rotational movement of the saddle.

This may appear to be a neat, clever, and satisfactory solution to the free-end saddle loading problem, especially in its most extreme form, the lower denture. However, there are problems:

- construction of the flexible component is difficult to control. Too light a structure and the force applied to the tissues is excessive, too heavy and the abutment tooth is too heavily loaded. The properties of the cast metal are subject to variability, for example casting flaws and inclusions
- fracture of the flexible connector can occur, from flexural fatigue or during cleaning. It may also become distorted during use or cleaning
- once damaged, repair may well not be possible, particularly with fracture
- from a more biological standpoint, alveolar resorption under the free-end saddle will gradually allow more flexure. This will progressively increase abutment tooth loading (which will also tend to increase the risk of fracture)
- rebasing will be difficult, since the flexible section will tend to bend during the development of the impression

Finally, there are available numerous prefabricated precision attachments which may be incorporated into the denture base, which can act both as hinges (simple or spring loaded) and saddle guides. This is outlined further in Chapter 3.10.

In summarizing the use of stress breakers, it has to be said that elegant though the concept is (and it has been described more fully in many texts) it is rarely advocated today. This may reflect the difficulties of being able to predict precisely how an individual design may work when subjected to occlusal loading of the saddle. The properties of the tissues and the materials of the denture base do not allow the clinician to make precise predictions as to how the saddle would move. Furthermore, even if a denture were to be made in this way, the physical characteristics of the supporting tissues may change over time, rendering the rationale for which the design was devised to be obsolete. Finally, other techniques (particularly the altered cast)

have generally been described more widely. Although an approach using stress breakers is now unlikely to be routinely used in clinical practice, it has been included to make you think about the particular problems that can occur in relation to a free-end saddle denture, and the approaches that have been used to solve these challenges. You might even come across a situation where you consider that this approach has specific advantages over the alternatives.

> ### Reminders
>
> Always remember that reducing the load applied to soft tissues is vital to their continued health and avoidance of increased alveolar remodelling:
>
> - fully extend the denture base
> - reduce the occlusal area
>
> Reducing the bucco-lingual dimension of the occlusal surface of lower chewing teeth gives further benefits:
>
> - the slope of the lower lingual flange is improved for muscular retention by the tongue
> - there is increased room available for the tongue to function, something which is very desirable if posterior teeth have been missing for some time and there is a degree of hypertrophy of the tongue, as it has had to take on some masticatory function
>
>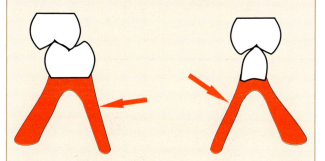
>
> Improved tongue space and angle of retentive muscle force
>
> The angle of the arrow on the right indicates the more beneficial downward (retentive) force exerted by the tongue on the lingual flange during function

Conclusions

The free-end saddle, particularly for the lower denture, raises specific challenges in relation to the provision of appropriate support. This primarily occurs because of the differences in potential displacement of the abutment tooth compared with the soft tissues directly under the saddle of the denture when a tooth and tissue supported prosthesis is used to replace the missing teeth. When considering the design of the denture in this situation some thought needs to be given to how the movement of the free-end saddle itself can be minimized during occlusal loading without causing damage to the underlying tissues.

Some points to remember

Numerous techniques have been developed in the attempt to solve the problem of the support differences provided by the teeth and the tissues for the free-end saddle case. Techniques such as:

- the RPI system
- tissue compression (altered cast)
- precision attachments (Chapter 3.10)
- reducing functional loads (decrease occlusal area, increase fitting area)

The shortened dental arch

Missing teeth do not always need to be replaced. Patients may be able to function effectively with a reduced dentition. The advantages and disadvantages of such an approach are considered.

We have previously posed the question as to whether it is necessary to replace missing teeth. The loss of an anterior tooth will usually cause the patient to seek treatment as they would find the aesthetics unacceptable. This may not be the case if one or more of the posterior teeth are lost. It might be expected that the loss of a number of teeth would compromise oral functions but, as shall be seen, this may not necessarily be true. The shortened dental arch concept evolved because it was recognized that reduced dentitions may be adequate for many patients and that the preservation of the teeth that remain was a more important objective than simply replacing teeth that were missing. Further, the quantity of chewing teeth we need nowadays, with modern softer diets, is not great so that the teeth are considerably under-exercised for good physiological health. In this chapter the potential advantages and disadvantages of the shortened dental arch will be explored.

What is a shortened dental arch?

The shortened dental arch has been defined as a reduced dentition primarily resulting from the loss of molar teeth. However the loss of premolar teeth could also contribute to this. The World Health Organization has set a goal for oral health as the retention of at least 20 natural teeth throughout adult life. However in the context of a shortened dental arch the number of teeth retained may be less important than the number of teeth that occlude with each other, thus allowing acceptable oral function. For example, a dentition in which all incisor, canine and premolar teeth are retained in the maxilla and mandible will mean that there are a number of pairs of occluding teeth. In contrast a dentition in which a mixture of molars and premolars have been lost may still retain 20 teeth but they may not all be occluding with one another. One might expect that mastication may be less efficient in the latter situation. The concept of the shortened dental arch involves directing treatment and resources to anterior and premolar teeth rather than molar teeth.

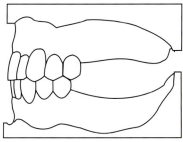

20 teeth — good occlusion

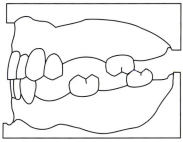

20 teeth — poor occlusion

When molar teeth are lost and not replaced, it is apparent that many patients are able to adapt their chewing and function with the occluding teeth that remain.

People with reduced dentitions may still have adequate masticatory ability. It would also seem that the number of occluding units is more important than the number of teeth present. The classical concept of the shortened dental arch involves the patient being able to function on 10 pairs of occluding units (i.e. a patient with incisors, canines, and premolars in the maxilla and mandible). It would seem that older people are more able to function in this way than patients who are younger. Indeed, it has even been suggested that patients over 70 years old could function on even fewer occluding units.

Patients may seek advice as to whether lost molar teeth should be replaced with a removable partial denture. The answer to this question primarily depends on the patient's own needs but a few points are worth considering on a general basis.

- The provision of partial dentures to replace molar teeth may not necessarily mean that there is an immediate increased masticatory efficiency. Patients may well have to develop new skills to use the prostheses effectively.

- If removable partial dentures are constructed the dentist should ensure that the patient understands the necessity for a high standard of oral and denture hygiene. It is critical that any prosthesis should not become a factor which contributes to further tooth loss in the future. This of course is true for any partial denture.

- In the case of mandibular free-end saddle dentures replacing molar teeth, it is believed that only a proportion of them are worn. The results of such studies have varied but the compliance may well be less than 50 per cent. The question would have to be asked as to whether this low take-up represents problems with denture design or simply that the patient finds it easier to function without the prosthesis.

Disadvantages of the shortened dental arch approach

Although there may be psychological effects on the patient in suggesting that teeth are not replaced, these would be difficult to measure objectively. However a patient for whom no treatment is recommended to replace missing posterior teeth would certainly need a full explanation of the reasons for this. Other potential

disadvantages of a shortened dental arch fall into two main categories.

- Excessive tooth wear of the remaining anterior teeth may result from a shortened dental arch. It might be expected that over time the remaining teeth would wear down more rapidly than if posterior teeth are present. Certainly patients may present with tooth wear in such situations. However the explanation may not be as simple as this. Patients may report parafunctional habits such as bruxism which may contribute to the attrition. Furthermore erosion of the teeth may be superimposed on damage from other causes. Nevertheless it would appear at least a theoretical possibility that patients with shortened dental arches are more susceptible to tooth wear. For this reason such patients should be monitored on a regular basis.

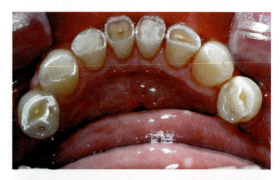
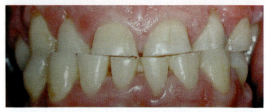

Anterior tooth wear which may be related in part to the loss of occluding posterior teeth

- With a shortened arch, it may mean that a patient who later needs posterior dental restoration due to further tooth loss, will present more of a problem with free-end saddles occupying the space previously available to the tongue. There may also have been a degree of hypertrophy of the tongue due to its taking on part of the masticatory function, or at least its inability to readapt to the space left free by the earlier extractions now occupied by the prosthesis.

- A greater susceptibility to temporomandibular joint dysfunction may also be associated with a shortened dental arch. It has been suggested that tooth loss which is not replaced may lead to abnormal loading on the temporomandibular joint and its associated musculature. However there would appear to be no compelling evidence to suggest that patients with reduced dentitions are actually more susceptible. Furthermore the replacement of molar teeth with free-end saddle partial dentures would not necessarily prevent the onset of temporomandibular joint dysfunction.

Conclusions

There are good reasons for accepting a shortened dental arch in a patient who reports that they have adequate teeth for satisfactory function. If a shortened dental arch situation is acceptable, it would nevertheless be wise to ensure that the patient is reviewed on a regular basis. A shortened dental arch may be unrealistic where tooth loss affects the appearance. Finally, each patient with missing posterior teeth should be assessed on an individual basis without any preconceived views from the dentist. Despite the general concepts that have been explored in this chapter, individual patients may be keenly aware of the loss of molar teeth and will seek restoration of the missing teeth with partial dentures. The dentist then needs to ensure that the prostheses are designed to be stable in function and will minimize the chances of further tooth loss.

Some points to remember

It may be quite acceptable for patients to function with reduced dentitions. The advantages and disadvantages of such an approach do, however, need to be considered carefully. It is important that the situation is monitored over time as patients' needs may change. Specific points to consider with this approach are:

- issues concerning the appearance
- the number of occluding teeth required for acceptable masticatory function
- the susceptibility of the remaining dentition to further disease

3.9 Partial dentures in conjunction with crowns

Consideration is given to the situation where teeth may require crowning and the advantages that this can give when designing a partial denture are discussed.

As discussed in Section 2, provision of a partial denture should not be embarked upon in isolation from other aspects of dental care, as teeth may need to be restored as an integral part of treatment. The dental history and examination will give the dentist the necessary information as to which teeth require attention. A treatment plan would usually be formulated which would involve the restoration of any carious teeth or failing restorations before the partial denture is constructed.

If it is necessary to crown any of the remaining teeth, there is an opportunity to construct them to give the best support, retention, and stability of the subsequent partial denture. This is essential if the crown is made for a tooth which is adjacent to a denture saddle.

Treatment planning and design of the denture

A full treatment plan should have been formulated from the history, examination, investigations, and an examination of the surveyed and articulated casts. The denture should be designed before any preparations for a crown are made.

Features of the crown that would be useful for a denture include:

- an occlusal rest seat
- a convex surface for an appropriately positioned clasp
- in some circumstances a guide plane
- an avoidance of undercut areas to reduce stagnation

In relation to the last bullet point, the exception to this would be the area of the crown for which a clasp tip can engage. In this case an undercut of the correct depth can be created in a planned position. However, to do this it is necessary to know what type of material would be used for the clasp arm and the appropriate way in which it will reach the undercut.

Procedure

The general procedure for designing a crown for an abutment tooth along with a partial denture is shown on a series of pictures from a model. Identical procedures would be used on a patient. The scenario shows how a crown and cobalt chromium based denture is constructed for a Kennedy II, modification 1 situation in which a crown is required on the premolar tooth adjacent to the bounded saddle.

- The treatment plan is formulated and the denture is designed. A metal ceramic crown is required for the abutment tooth shown by the arrow. It is planned to incorporate specific features into the crown that will be of benefit for the partial denture (see Appendix 1 for a suggested design proforma).

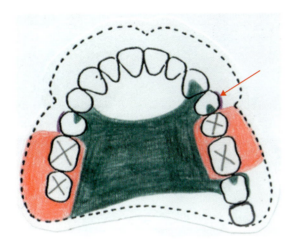

The original denture design, the arrow indicates
the tooth that requires a crown

- If required a guide plane is made on the abutment
tooth at the opposite end of the saddle (in this case the
molar tooth). This will be made to coincide with the path
of insertion of the denture.

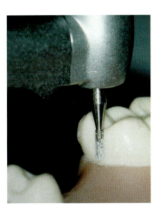

Preparation of a guide plane on the abutment tooth
at the other end of the saddle from the crown

- The crown preparation is carried out. It should be
noted that a rest seat has been incorporated into the
occlusal surface of the crown preparation (to allow
enough thickness for it to be reproduced in the surface of the crown) on the distal aspect adjacent to the
saddle. After the preparation is complete an impression is recorded.

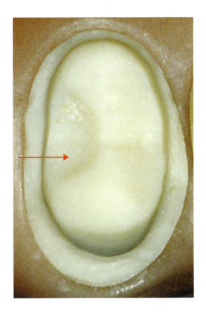

Completed crown preparation, the occlusal
rest seat is indicated by the arrow

- The crown is formed with features to optimize the fit
of the partial denture. In these illustrations it can be seen
that the distal surface of the crown is shaped so that it
is parallel with the guide plane on the abutment tooth
at the opposite end of the saddle.

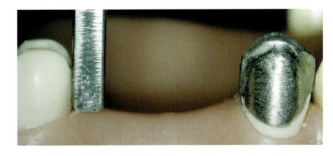

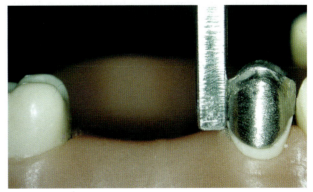

The surveyor is used to make the crown
with the correct guide plane

• An occlusal rest seat has been incorporated into the crown on the distal aspect of the tooth. This will allow an occlusal rest on the prosthesis to engage precisely.

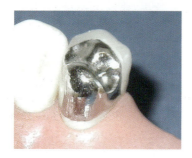

The completed metal ceramic crown

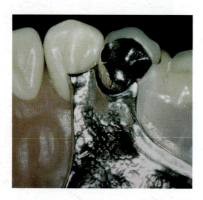

The fit of the denture around the crown

• The metallic parts of the crown are constructed so that stagnation undercuts are avoided. On the buccal aspect of the tooth a convex surface has been created in the ceramic (arrowed). The depth of the undercut (0.75 mm) is suited to the very flexible acetyl-resin tooth coloured clasp employed in this particular design.

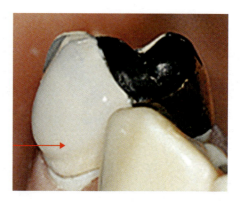

The arrow indicates where the convex bulbosity has been positioned on the ceramic

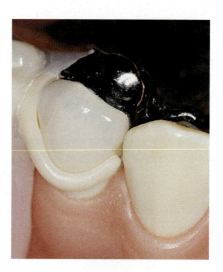

Acetyl-resin clasp engaging the undercut

• The final denture is made to the original design.

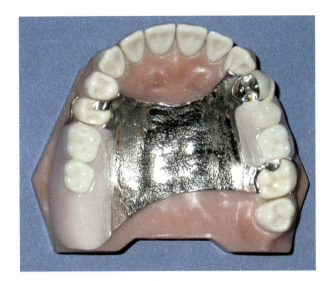

Denture made to the original design

Precision attachments

There are a wide variety of prefabricated precision-made attachments which can be incorporated into or on to (intra or extra coronal) a crown during its manufacture. These are to aid in the support and/or retention of a prosthesis (see Chapter 3.10).

Conclusions

In many situations dentures have to be made around crowns that are already present in the mouth. In these cases the partial denture has to be planned in the same way as for the other natural teeth. However where a crown is required as part of the overall treatment plan, there is scope to design the crown to suit the needs of the partial denture. Good communication between the dentist and dental technician is essential so that each member of the team understands exactly what is required.

Some points to remember

If a crown is required on an abutment tooth the dentist has an ideal opportunity to incorporate features which will optimize the support, retention and stability of the partial denture. It is critical therefore, that the denture design is formulated before the crown is prepared. Close liaison between the dentist and the technicians involved in the making of the crown and partial denture is needed. Specific points to consider in crown design are:

• appropriately sited and shaped occlusal rest seats
• appropriately sited and shaped bulbosities so that optimally designed clasps can be incorporated in the partial denture
• appropriately sited guide planes
• appropriately shaped surfaces to avoid stagnation where a denture is in contact with it

3.10 Some mechanical complexities

Some examples of more complex techniques developed to attempt to overcome difficulties in gaining support and/or retention are as follows:

- precision attachments
- swinglock
- disjunct denture
- two-part dentures

Precision attachments

Precision attachments can be incorporated into crowns and dentures so that the support, retention, and stability can be enhanced. There are many different types of attachment and it is not within the remit of this text to consider these in detail (see Further reading). The principle of their use is that an attachment is incorporated into a crown which has a companion component in the prosthesis to which it can locate when the denture is inserted. There are some specific issues arising from their use.

- High forces can be generated on the crown from occlusal loading of the saddle. It is critical that the underlying tooth structure can withstand these and that the periodontal attachment is not overloaded.

- It is desirable that the tooth carrying the attachment should be loaded down its long axis. A precision attachment on an overdenture abutment as shown in Chapter 3.6 would allow optimum loading. Great care should be taken in the use of extra-coronal attachments as the loading will take place principally on one side of the tooth (and periodontium).

- The standard of oral hygiene should be very high indeed. There are inevitable areas of stagnation around attachments in which plaque can accumulate. The patient needs to be very effective in plaque removal.

- As mechanical components such as springs form part of some attachments, it is inevitable that maintenance and even replacement of part of the components will be required from time to time.

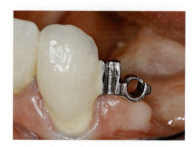

Coronal part

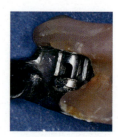

Saddle part

A precision lock between the tooth- and the tissue-supported denture parts

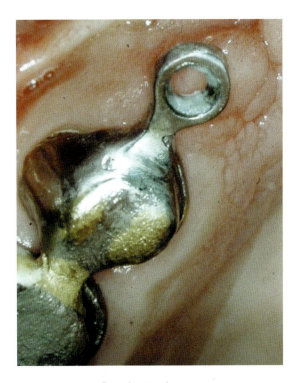

Female attachment

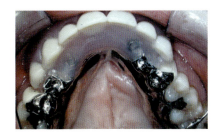

Fitted denture

The denture retained by precision attachments
joining it to tooth preparations

The swinglock denture

The swinglock denture has been used to restore arches in
which there are a very small number of teeth remaining
leading to significant retention and stability problems.
The denture has an additional locking bar connected to
a hinge. This allows part of the prosthesis to engage the
teeth and their undercuts from the labial aspect, and they
are typically used for large free-end saddles of lower dentures.
The posterior part is essentially conventional, with such
tooth and tissue support as is available.

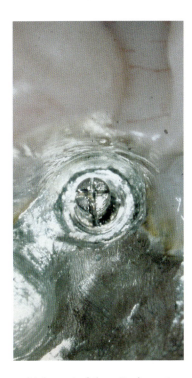

Male part of the attachment

The female part is attached to the part fixed to the tooth
restorations, the male part to the prosthesis

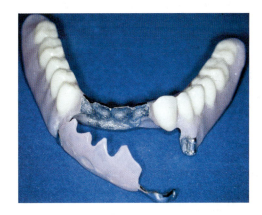

Labial flange in the open position

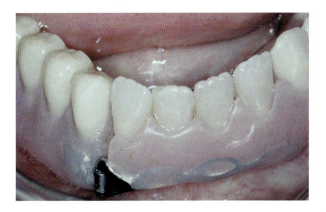

Hinge closed

Advantages

- The swinglock denture will engage potentially deep and otherwise inaccessible labial undercuts.
- Retention is very good.
- Aesthetics are improved if there is some unsightly gingival recession.

Disadvantages

- The teeth will be gripped tightly from the denture components on the lingual and labial aspects. Occlusal loading of the saddle will therefore tend to apply potentially damaging forces to the teeth that remain. This situation will be exacerbated if there is alveolar resorption in the saddle areas. The technique would be contraindicated in patients in which the remaining teeth have periodontal disease.
- As much of the tooth surfaces and gingival tissues are covered by the prosthesis, this renders them particularly susceptible to the effects of plaque. If the patient cannot maintain exemplary levels of plaque control, caries or periodontal disease can occur.
- The locking catch is difficult to rectify when worn or distorted.
- Patient tolerance of the labial component can be poor because it can feel intrusive.
- Although of great assistance with retention, the system does not help with support.

The authors advise great caution in the use of swing-lock dentures. Although they can result in enhanced stability of the prosthesis, any advantage is rapidly lost if further disease results either from unwanted mechanical effects during occlusal loading or because the patient does not clean the mouth and dentures effectively.

The disjunct denture

Disjunct dentures have been used when the remaining (usually anterior) teeth are of poor prognosis and offer inadequate support. Typically, they are used when there are two lower free-end saddles. It consists of two separate parts which are linked together into one unit. A tooth-borne part provides splinting for the remaining teeth and a means of retention for the mucosa-borne part. The two parts of the denture are attached to each other by a sliding pin and slot mechanism. This permits the saddles to move vertically during occlusal loading. The disjunction

between the two parts of the denture may make it more comfortable to wear than a conventional single part prosthesis. As the tooth-borne part of the prosthesis is on teeth that have lost periodontal support, there is a danger of further periodontal attachment loss, particularly if the oral hygiene is inadequate. They are not widely used.

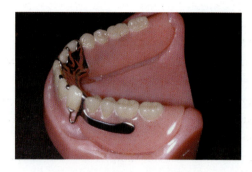

The denture is in two independent parts, one is tooth supported, the other tissue supported. However, although loosely connected they cannot be separated.

The tooth supported part only contributes retention to the tissue supported part.

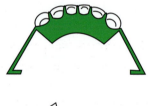

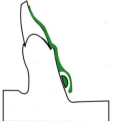

Bar protected by skirt

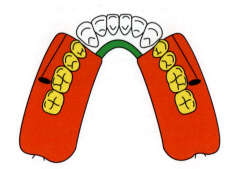

Tooth supported extensions connect with, and slide within, vertical slots on the tissue supported part

The posterior portion, usually acrylic saddles joined by a cast metal bar, is designed to be tissue supported and has no rests or clasps. It is retained and stabilized by the anterior tooth supported splinting component.

Advantages

- Large posterior saddles do not rely on support from abutment teeth (which may not be in good order themselves).
- The remaining teeth can be splinted together to act as a single unit during incision.
- In function, vertical movement of the tissue supported part is permitted, without levering the anterior section which only provides retention.
- With alveolar remodelling, the posterior part can sink to a considerable degree without placing leverage on to the anterior component, due to the length of the slide.
- Gum 'stripping' is avoided by the lingual bar being clear of the gingival margins and a protective skirt (cast into the anterior part) around the distal side of the teeth adjacent to the tissue supported saddles.

Disadvantages

- More complex to construct and maintain.
- Potential for bone resorption from the tissue supported saddles.
- Patient resistance to the bulk of the denture (lingually due to the lingual bar and its covering skirt).

The sectional dentures (two-part)

Sectional dentures are occasionally of use when replacing small saddles. The principle of using these is that the prosthesis is made in two parts which allows engagement of opposing undercuts that would normally act as interferences to the seating of a denture. Many different designs have been described. Typically such dentures are made for a Kennedy III where there are opposing mesial and distal undercuts, for instance distally on a premolar and mesially on a molar. The two parts of the denture need to be locked together. They can be separate components, one part fitting from the lingual aspect and the other from the buccal aspect, the two parts can then be bolted together.

Alternatively the two components can be attached to each other by means of a hinge and lock, so that the two parts of the prosthesis can then be swung into position and bolted together. The advantage of these dentures is that they can be made with minimal tissue coverage. As the components are bolted together there is little danger of them moving or becoming displaced during function. A unilateral denture should never be made unless it can be locked into position without the possibility of it being displaced, by function or any other means, for it could be swallowed or even worse inhaled.

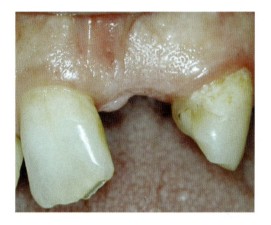

For a sectional denture deep mesial and distal undercuts are essential for retention, as they are engaged by the denture base which inserts from the labial and palatal directions

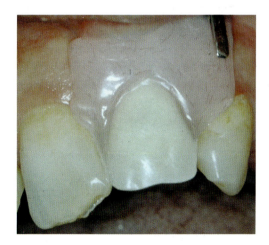

The locking bolt is high in the sulcus (unobtrusive) and the interdental papillae restored

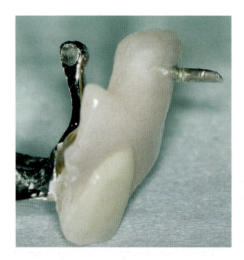

The hinge is in the open position, note the hole in the top of the metal part for the locking bolt

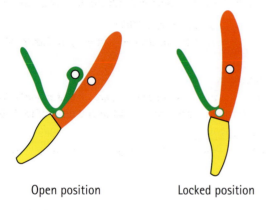

Open position   Locked position

The bolt for locking cannot be shown as it lies at a right angle to the section of the denture illustrated, and passes through the holes in the flange and denture when locked (the lower hole is part of the hinge)

Advantages

- Locking into place prevents movement or displacement.
- Avoids the need for a connector to other regions.
- Does not need extensive tooth preparation associated with conventional bridgework.

Disadvantages

- The bolts may loosen over time due to wear of the metal making the prosthesis much less secure.

- Risks to local oral health unless the patient can be fully relied upon to remove the appliance regularly and frequently for cleaning (and meticulous oral hygiene in the area is also required).
- Manual dexterity required for insertion and removal.
- Largely superseded by adhesive bridgework (with minimal tooth preparation) or implants.
- A highly skilled technician is required for the fabrication of the appliance.

Conclusions

We hope that, from this chapter you have grasped the basic ideas behind these designs. All have involved the following:

- clinical judgement
- patient selection
- clinical skill
- technical expertise

followed by exemplary patient self-care and professional recall and review.

For more extensive study, we recommend recourse to the reading list we have provided, together with consultation of past and current literature. Perhaps this is the best possible note on which to end—continuing professional development.

Some points to remember

Many ingenious devices have been, and are yet to be, developed to improve or refine the aesthetics and function of partial dentures, mainly through striving to gain the optimum support, retention, and aesthetics. Some of the general principles involved when using these devices are as follows:

- do not overload the underlying tooth structure or periodontal attachment
- a high standard of oral hygiene must be maintained
- there is a need to design the prostheses so that components can be maintained or replaced easily if required

Further reading

The following texts will be of interest to readers who wish to explore further aspects of treatment planning and design as well as the procedures that are used in the construction of partial dentures.

Alan B. Carr, Glen P. McGivney, and David T. Brown
McCracken's Removable Partial Prosthodontics, 11th edn, St Louis: Mosby, 2005.

J. Fraser McCord, Alan A. Grant, Callum C. Youngson, Roger M. Watson, and David M. Davis
Missing Teeth: A Guide to Treatment Options, Edinburgh: Churchill Livingstone, 2003.

Rodney D. Phoenix, David R. Cagna, and Charles F. DeFreest
Stewart's Clinical Removable Partial Prosthodontics, 3rd edn, London: Quintessence, 2003.

Bengt Öwall, Arnd F. Käyser, and Gunnar E. Carlsson
Prosthodontics: Principles and Management Strategies, London: Mosby-Wolfe, 1996.

Sybille K. Lechner and A.R. MacGregor
Removable Partial Prosthodontics: A Case-oriented Manual of Treatment Planning, London: Wolfe, 1994.

John C. Davenport, Robin M. Basker, John R. Heath, James P. Ralph, and Per-Olof Glantz
A Clinical Guide to Removable Partial Dentures: The Assessment and Treatment of Patients Requiring RPDs, London: British Dental Association, 2000.

John C. Davenport, Robin M. Basker, John R. Heath, James P. Ralph, and Per-Olof Glantz
A Clinical Guide to Removable Partial Denture Design, London: British Dental Association, 2000.

Russell J. Stratton and Frank J. Wiebelt
An Atlas of Removable Partial Denture Design, London: Quintessence Books, 1988.

N.J.A. Jepson
Removable Partial Dentures. Quintessentials of Dental Practice, Editor-in-Chief Nairn H.R. Wilson. London: Quintessence Publishing Company, 2004.

A. Damien Walmsley, Trevor F. Walsh, F.J. Trevor Burke, Adrian C.C. Shortall, Philip J. Lumley, and Richard Hayes-Hall
Restorative Dentistry, Edinburgh: Churchill Livingstone, 2002.

Joseph E. Grasso and Ernest L. Miller
Removable Partial Prosthodontics, 3rd edn, St. Louis: Mosby, 1991.

Gareth Jenkins
Precision Attachments—A Link to Successful Restorative Treatment, Illinois: Quintessence Publishing Company Ltd, 1999.

Ejvind Budtz-Jorgensen
Prosthodontics for the Elderly, Illinois: Quintessence Publishing Company Ltd, 1999.

Appendix 1

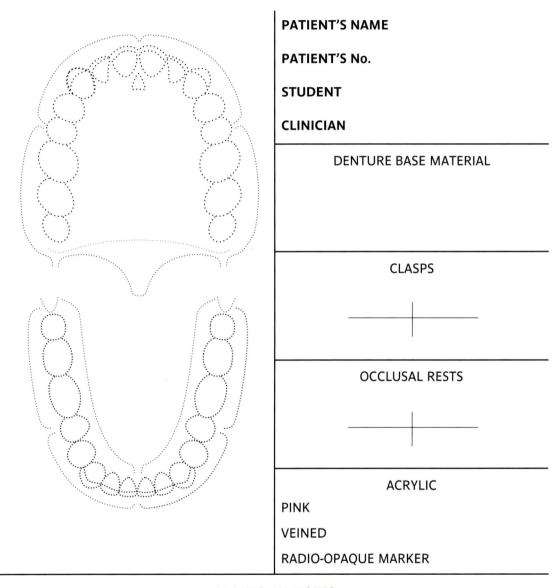

PATIENT'S NAME

PATIENT'S No.

STUDENT

CLINICIAN

DENTURE BASE MATERIAL

CLASPS

OCCLUSAL RESTS

ACRYLIC

PINK

VEINED

RADIO-OPAQUE MARKER

ADDITIONAL NOTES

Index

Page entries for illustrations appear in **bold** type
Page entries for headings which also have subheadings refer only to general aspects of that topic.

A

abrasion 91, **92**
acrylic resin denture bases 41, 78
additions to dentures 96, 98
  attachment of additional teeth 97/**97**
  loss of essential components due to extraction 96
  overdentures 97
  timing of extractions 96
aesthetic considerations 3, 4, 5
  and cast surveying 17, 22, 27
  overdentures 113/**113**
  tooth loss 3
ageing dentition, design of dentures 91, 94; *see also* residual dentition
  clinical assessment 92
  connector selection 94
  crown-root ratio 92
  design sequence for healthy dentition 93–94, **94**
  manageing neglected dentition 95
  retention 94
  saddle location/design 93
  gingival recession 92–93, **93**
  root exposure/root caries 93/**93**, 94
  tooth wear 91, **92**, 92–93
  undercut zones 92, **93**, 94
Altered Cast Technique 120, **121**
alveolar remodelling 31, 111/**111**, 116, 120, 123
analysing rods 26/**26**, 47
anterior
  bars **74**, 78
  plates **74**
  saddles, labial flanges 82/**82**
articulated study casts 69–70, **69**

cast surveying 70
design 71
record blocks 69, 70
attrition 91, **92**

B

badly damaged *see* neglected dentition; *see also* caries; difficult dentitions; tooth wear
bars; *see also* rigid connectors
  anterior 35/**35**, **74**, 78
  buccal 39/**39**
  dental 38/**38**, 75
  lingual 36, 37–38, **37**
  lingual bar with minor connector 38–39/**39**
  middle 35/**35**, **74**
  palatal 35/**35**, 78
  posterior 35/**35**, **74**
bilateral free-end saddles 11, **12–16**; *see also* class I dentures
bone remodelling 31, 111/**111**, 116, 120, 123
bounded saddles *see* class III dentures
bracing/bracing action 46/**46**
bridges 5, 82
  patient preferences 67
buccal bars 39/**39**

C

cantilevered support *see* indirect support
caries
  root 93/**93**, 94, 114
  susceptibility to 89
cast surveying 17–20, 27, 42; *see also* clasps; denture bases; undercuts
  aesthetic considerations 17, 22, 27
  articulated study casts 70
  construction of cast surveyor 17/**17**
  free-end saddle 25

insertional interferences 17/**17**
  lingual plates 25
  non-undercut area 18
  survey line 18
  tissue/denture blend 17, 22, 27
cingulum rests 78
clasps
  clasp/rest combinations 54–55
  design examples 55–57, **55**, **56**, **57**
  extended arm 44/**44**
  gingivally approaching/roach 42/**42**, 44–45, **44**, **45**
  indirect retention 54–55/**54**
  occlusally approaching 42/**42**, 44/**44**
  positioning 48–50, **48**, **49**, **50**
  recurved arm 44/**44**
  surveying 17, 19–20/**20**, 21, 22
  tips 48, 49, 50
  trip action 42–43/**43**
  undercuts/undercut areas 23, 24, 27
class I/II dentures, designing for 77, 81, 119, 123/**123**, 124
  Altered Cast Technique 120, **121**
  cast surveying 25
  combined support/retention (RPI) system 79–80, **80**
  connector selection 78
  definitions 11
  flexible connectors 120, 121–123, **121**, **122**
  indirect retention 78–79, **78**, **79**
  other management options 120
  review of provisional design 80–81
  saddle design methods 77
  support 77–78, **77**, 119–120, 124

watch out for gum stripping 77
  tissue displacement (compression) whilst taking impressions 120–121, **121**
class III dentures, designing for 73, 76
  connector selection 73–75, **74**, **75**
  definition 11
  lower dentures **75**
  oral hygiene considerations/implications 73, 75, 76
  retention, direct/indirect 75–76, **76**
  review of provisional design 76
  saddle design examples 73/**73**
  support 73
  upper dentures **74**
class IV dentures, designing for 82, 88
  labial flange for anterior saddles 82/**82**
  lower denture connectors 84
  retention 84–85, **84**, **85**
  review of provisional design 86/**86**
  saddle design 85–86, **85**
  saddle design for a few missing teeth 82/**82**
  support for short anterior saddle 83/**83**
  temporary replacement of a few teeth 87/**87**
  temporary replacement of large anterior saddle 87
  upper denture connectors 83/**83**
classification 11, 16; *see also* class I/II; class III; class IV dentures; Kennedy classification
cobalt chromium based denture bases 41
comfort considerations 3, 4
composite resin 45/**45**

vertical/horizontal plane
20/**20**
unilateral free-end saddles
12/**12–16**; *see also* class II
dentures